Osteoporosis Unlocked:
Natural Strategies for a Healthier, Stronger You

Dr. John Stephen, PT, PPD, Cert.MDT, COMT.

This book is dedicated to my uncle, Dr. Jacob John, PhD (Australia), whose inspiration led me to pursue further education and aid those in need.

Table of Contents

About The Author

John Stephen PT, PPD, Cert. MDT, COMPT

Clinic Director for Rehab Specialists

John is a master clinician (PT) specializing in advanced Orthopedic manual techniques and is a certified orthopedic manual therapist. He received his Post-Professional Clinical Doctorate in 2006 with a concentration in advanced Orthopedics. He graduated as a physiotherapist in the early 90s and has over 30 years of clinical expertise. Dr. Stephen is also an APTA-certified clinical instructor. With extensive experience in treating back and neck pain with radiating symptoms, he has an active interest in sharing his expertise through mentoring and has taught numerous courses. Dr. Stephen is certified in the McKenzie method and spinal manipulative therapy and has extensive Orthopedic manual training in extremities and the spine. He has worked with area surgeons and physicians to develop evidence-based protocols for orthopedic, neuro-surgical, and sports medicine conditions. Dr. Stephen's research interests include osteoporosis, spine, nerve injuries, and interventions for peripheral neuropathy, and he has successfully developed an evidence-based protocol for treating peripheral neuropathy. Additionally, Dr. Stephen is the author of *Peripheral Neuropathy: A Patient's Guide to Self-Management,* available on Amazon.

Acknowledgments

I would like to give a sincere thank you to my family. Without their love and support, this book would not be possible. I want to thank my niece, Shinu Sam, for her consultation and contribution to the nutritional information presented in this book.

The exercise portion of this book was greatly enhanced, thanks to the help and expertise of my co-workers, Megan Bly, PT, DPT, and Allyson Lowis, DPT, COMT.

I would like to thank my co-workers, Alicia Marsh, DPT, COMT, Brindlea Peterson, Brenton Rozycki, DPT, COMT, and Devin Uhrich, for their photographic contributions.

Thank you to Dr. Jeff Coppinger, MD, Andy Fate, MSPT, COMT, MBA, and Dr. Steven Osterhout, DC, CCN, for sharing their knowledge and expertise in this book's medical and nutritional sections.

I want to thank everyone who helped proofread the book, specifically Brindlea Peterson, for helping to make this book as accessible and easy to read as possible.

Finally, I want to express my sincere gratitude to my Rehab Specialist's family for their support and dedication to bettering the lives of our patients.

Introduction

Hi, my name is Dr. John Stephen, and I am a physical therapist, credentialed clinical instructor, and mentor. Over the past 30 years, I have treated more than 15,000 patients of different age groups and with various diagnoses, preventing many from undergoing surgery. I have extensive experience and multiple specializations in spinal health (including certifications and degrees from the United States, India, Ireland, and Australia) and a keen interest in helping those affected by osteoporosis.

My goal is to help you achieve the best health outcomes by creating treatment plans that include simple, realistic, and effective home exercises – all based on clinically proven research studies and years of expert experience.

For the past 30 years, I have been dedicated to researching and implementing effective strategies. I can say with certainty that I love what I do! I am excited to help you along your healing journey. Let's get started!

How To Use This Book

Did you know that as we age, our bone health decreases? A reduction in bone mass leads to osteoporosis, which, in turn, results in frequent falls, injuries, and fractures. Following a healthy diet and exercise plan is the most effective solution to safeguard your bone health.

The main goal of the book, ***Osteoporosis Unlocked: Natural Strategies for a Healthier, Stronger You,*** is to stop bone loss and effectively rebuild your bone health from the comfort of your home. This book will help you understand your diagnoses while offering tips, recommendations, and examples of nutrition plans and easy and safe at-home exercises, all with clear instructions and **all** designed based on various clinically proven and research-based scientific studies.

Plan Components

In this book, you will learn:

- How to manage life with osteoporosis

- How to transform your life after you've been diagnosed with osteoporosis through a natural approach to a healthy, improved, and positive lifestyle

- How to implement dietary guidelines to help manage osteoporosis and its related side effects

- How to perform carefully selected, simple, and clinically proven at-home exercises to strengthen your body and help you feel your best

- How to prevent frequent falls and fractures to hip, spine, and wrist bones

- How to follow a whole-body, comprehensive plan that will set you up for long-term improved bone health.

- How to correct and maintain good posture.

Are you ready to begin your journey toward a happier, healthier lifestyle? By following the guidelines in this book, you will be well on your way to improving both your quality of life and your long-term bone health. Get ready to enjoy your transformation.

Happy reading!

Disclaimer

The information provided here is not intended to replace the doctor's recommendations. If you are new to exercise, I strongly recommend you first talk to your healthcare provider or a specialist who would recommend you for bone density and other required physical assessment tests to identify your bone health condition. Based on your results the healthcare provider would suggest the safest and appropriate exercises. I also recommend you stop doing exercises if you experience any pain or discomfort. Also, this booklet takes no responsibility for any health issues that arise from following the plans provided.

Chapter 1

Life With Osteoporosis

Living with osteoporosis can often cause a tough time. Some develop a fear of frequent falls and fractures, whereas others feel grateful to receive an early diagnosis. Whether you or a loved one has been diagnosed with Osteoporosis, we are here to help you learn how to lessen bone loss and maintain bone health.

Understanding Osteoporosis

Osteoporosis (which means 'porous bone') is a highly prevalent yet silent epidemic that affects the bone density of an individual. This bone disorder develops with increased age and occurs when there is a quick loss of bone minerals (such as calcium) that exceeds the body's capability to replace them. As a result, the bones become weak and brittle, often leading to hip, wrist, or spine fractures. You may never know that you have osteoporosis until your bones are broken! For those with osteoporosis, even a small action, such as sneezing, can lead to fragility fractures, which are indeed both painful and serious.

What Causes It

Bones are renewed through constant remodeling and repair processes. During the younger ages, bone growth occurs quickly with healthy levels of bone mass and slows down with increased age. For osteoporosis patients, bone thinning occurs at such a pace that the bone loss exceeds the bone production. As a result, bones become weak and fragile with less bone density, thereby making the patient susceptible to fractures in their hip, wrist, and spine. Causes of osteoporosis include reduced levels of estrogen in females, low testosterone in males, calcium and/or vitamin D deficiencies, a sedentary lifestyle, thyroid conditions, smoking, excessive alcohol intake, the use of certain medications, and some underlying medical conditions.

Risk factors for osteoporosis are categorized into non-modifiable factors and modifiable factors. The non-modifiable risk factors are risks that cannot be prevented or modified. They are primarily responsible for the onset of osteoporosis. They can include factors such as advancing age, gender (females are more likely to suffer from osteoporosis than males), family history, skeletal disorders, usage of certain medications, a history of endocrine disorders, fractures, previous hysterectomies in females, and hypogonadism in males. Modifiable, or changeable, risk factors are those factors that can be improved by you and your physician. Some modifiable risk factors include physical inactivity, poor nutrition, eating disorders, and reduced body weight.

Effects On Body And Mind

Osteoporosis affects both the body and mind of a person in various ways and is widely linked with various disabilities and high mortality rates. The most common ailments that are associated with osteoporosis are Paget's disease of the bones, depression, spinal compression fractures and deformities, bone cancer, cardiac failure, and osteoarthritis.

Some of the typical early physical symptoms of bone loss include receding gums, brittle fingernails, and weak grip strength. Other physical symptoms of osteoporosis that develop at its later stages can include stooped posture, abnormal curving of the spine, back pain, and bone fractures.

The chronic stress put on the body because of osteoporosis can often cause long-term mental stress, resulting in depression and anxiety disorders. Without the proper treatment and support system, it is easy for people with osteoporosis to develop a poor quality of living along with various behavioral changes and altered sleep patterns. They may develop a fear of falling or fractures which can lead to feelings of melancholy, helplessness, sudden awareness of increased age/mortality, a lack of confidence, low self-esteem, reduced self-image, loss of independence, and a decreased desire to engage in physical activities. The signs and symptoms of osteoporosis are known to differ in each individual based on their age, gender, ethnicity, health conditions, and family background.

Knowing Your Bone Mineral Density

Bone Mineral Density (BMD), or bone density, refers to the inorganic content of bone minerals, which is approximately 65% hydroxyapatite (calcium and phosphorous). Osteoporosis can be diagnosed by testing for BMD even before the breakage of bone takes place. The test is accurate, painless, and key in determining bone health and quality. A test known as the Central Dual-Energy X-ray Absorptiometry is one of the most popular and widely used BMD tests. According to the National Osteoporosis Foundation (NOF), a BMD test is recommended for all women aged 65 and above and for all men aged 70 and above, irrespective of the presence or absence of risk factors. The test is performed after obtaining a prescription/referral from a healthcare professional. The indicators that may prompt your physician to run a BMD test include a decrease in height, fragility fractures, an estrogen deficiency in females, long-term usage of steroid medications, bone marrow or organ transplants, and signs of hormonal imbalances.

The test results of the BMD assessment are reported with a T-score value and a Z-score value. The T-score value is calculated by comparing the BMD values of the patient with the values of a healthy 30-year-old adult. The lower the value of the T-score, the lower the patient's bone density. Z-score values are derived by comparing the value of the patient with that of a healthy individual of the same age as the patient and are used to evaluate BMD among children and young adults. In addition to running a BMD assessment, your doctor may also order laboratory tests that can help evaluate your rate of bone loss and bone production (known as "bone turnover markers" or "biochemical markers").

T-Score Readings And Density Indications

Score	Diagnosis
-1.0 or above	Normal
-1.0 to -2.5	Low bone density
-2.5 or below	Osteoporosis

Who is most likely to develop osteoporosis? Based on the 2010 data, NOF estimated that out of the 54 million people in America, 10.2 million were diagnosed with osteoporosis. Of those diagnosed, 80 percent were found to be women. One in every two women aged 50 and above and one in every four men aged 50 and above are diagnosed with low bone mass and/or osteoporosis. People with autoimmune disorders such as Rheumatoid Arthritis, Lupus, Multiple Sclerosis, and Ankylosing Spondylitis are more prone to the disease.

Females are more frequently affected than males because they typically have thinner bones than males. Additionally, the decrease in estrogen production that occurs post-menopause contributes to increased diagnoses. The condition differs among females based on age and ethnicity. It is estimated that 20% of Caucasian women, 5% of African American women, 20% of Asian-American women, and 10% of Latinas aged 50 and above are more susceptible to the disease. However, no matter what age group you're in or what lifestyle habits you follow, you are never too old or too young to take care of and preserve your bone health. With the right diet and exercise plan, you can be sure to regain and sustain your bone strength.

Current Treatments

While there is currently no cure for osteoporosis, there are various treatments available to stop or reverse bone loss, ranging from medications and supplements to physical therapy. The treatments available slow down the process of bone loss and strengthen bone health. By following the right approach and making healthy lifestyle choices, you can easily improve your osteoporosis symptoms.

Common Medications To Consider

Treating osteoporosis without using any form of medication is challenging. This is because the most common and effective medications (such as bisphosphonate drugs, dietary and vitamin supplements, monoclonal antibody medications, hormonal therapy, and certain bone-building medications) are found to increase bone density by preventing bone loss.

Supplements – Are They Worth It?

Nutrients present in food are known to play a great role in maintaining the strength and health of the bones. The intake of a well-balanced diet is known to nourish bone health whereas a diet that lacks calcium, vitamin D, and other essential nutrients often leads to poor bone health. More often than not, nutritional supplements are found to be useful for bone health. Your doctor may recommend supplements in order to compensate for the deficiency of essential bone nutrients that are normally obtained through the intake of a well-balanced diet. These supplements can enhance a well-balanced diet while supporting bone health and preventing further bone loss. Calcium, Vitamin D, Magnesium, Vitamin K, and Lycopene are the most vital nutrients that are essential for people diagnosed with osteoporosis to ingest. These nutrients can ease inflammation, strengthen bones, and prevent further bone loss. Among these essential supplements for osteoporosis prevention, calcium, and vitamin D have been proven to be the most effective supplements for preventing bone loss and maintaining the health of bones.

Even though these nutritional supplements have proven to be effective for bone health, in some cases, it is found that certain health conditions (such as lactose intolerance or digestive diseases) may affect the ability of the body to filter these essential nutrients. Additionally, certain substances should be avoided, such as caffeine, alcohol, carbonated drinks, and salt. Therefore, it is always important to talk with your doctor before taking supplements to make sure that they are the right ones for you.

How Physical Therapy Helps

Physical therapy plays an effective and important role in treating and managing pain associated with osteoporosis and bone fractures and can help you feel your best by providing pain management strategies and ways to improve your balance and posture. Physical therapy often enhances one's ability to regain self-confidence and manage pain associated with osteoporosis and strength of bones and muscles, thereby lessening the risk of frequent falls and associated bone fractures.

Low Back Pain In Osteoporosis

1. **Strengthening Muscles: Specific exercises** can help **strengthen the muscles** that support the spine. By targeting the anti-gravity muscles like the lumbar paraspinals, quadriceps, and gluteals, they help stabilize the spine well. When your core muscles are more robust, they make a corset around your spine. A trained physical therapist could help design a program specific to your needs.

2. **Posture and Balance: Practices like gentle tai chi and yoga,** which focus on **posture and balance**, can be particularly helpful for individuals with osteoporosis. Improved posture will help reduce the stress on the spine and other joints of the body.

3. **Flexibility and Mobility**: **Stretching exercises** are essential for maintaining joint mobility and preventing muscle spasms and low back pain.

4. **Pain Management**: Physical therapists often use heat or cold modalities and gentle mobilization techniques to reduce pain in addition to pain medications.

Remember that while exercise is beneficial, safety is paramount. Individuals with spine osteoporosis should avoid forceful twisting movements, high-impact exercises, and activities that carry a risk of fractures. Always consult with a spine physical therapist to tailor an exercise program that suits your specific needs and limitations.

To begin your healing journey, you will likely receive a specially tailored treatment plan from your physical therapist based on your age, gender, bone health, and fracture risk. This will also include an appropriate exercise plan with fall prevention education, weight-bearing exercises, balance activities, strength training, pain relief measures, and healthy lifestyle advice to prevent your bones from further thinning while improving your balance and bone strength. Weight-bearing exercises that involve walking and other low-impact exercises are found to be very effective in preventing the loss of bone mass caused by osteoporosis.

Talking With Your Doctor

It is important for osteoporosis patients to have regular check-ups with their doctors to measure their progress, check their current status, and discuss any concerns they may have. It is essential to let your doctor know about your family history, medical history, current medications (even over-the-counter medications, herbal remedies, and/or supplements), and any nutritional supplements that you currently use or have used to treat various ailments and health conditions in the past. Details of your diet plan, treatment of any chronic conditions, and complete surgical history should also be discussed with your doctor during the visit. Habits such as smoking and alcohol intake are also considered essential criteria to mention while talking with your doctor.

A New Way To Heal

The primary goal of every treatment plan is to alleviate pain and promote quick healing. With osteoporosis, even though various methods have proven to be very effective, one of the best things you can do to mitigate pain and promote effective bone health is to adopt a healthy diet.

Eating To Heal

The food we consume doesn't just leave a pleasant taste in our mouths but is also known to impact our overall health on various levels. Eating a clean diet and adopting a healthy lifestyle are known to lessen the length of recovery for various health conditions. This is because food with high-quality nutrients is required for effective healing. Therefore, it is essential to pause and think about our food choices and our relationship with food to heal and maintain a healthy lifestyle.

Strong bones are built through a balanced and healthy diet and, from an early age, the food we eat can either help to maintain or to deteriorate our bone health throughout our entire lives. A balanced diet rich in calcium and vitamin D is essential for maintaining the strength and health of bones and enhancing the prevention of bone loss. In addition to calcium and vitamin D, a healthy meal rich in protein, vitamin C, iron, magnesium, and potassium can be useful in enhancing bone health in patients with osteoporosis. A detailed description of the importance of a balanced diet (along with some easy-to-follow examples) is provided in Chapter 2.

Managing Sleep And Stress

Stress management and the cultivation of good sleep are known to play a vital part in managing osteoporosis. Many osteoporosis patients constantly worry about falling, which causes increased stress levels and often results in calcium depletion. Similarly, not getting enough sleep (or sleeping poorly) impacts the musculoskeletal system and affects bone mineral density by causing imbalances in the bone remodeling process. As a result, the risk of osteoporosis increases. Therefore, stress relief strategies and proper sleep patterns are essential for rejuvenation and bone strengthening in osteoporosis patients.

Embracing Exercise

Your overall physical and mental health may improve by embracing the right exercise program. According to NOF, patients with a positive attitude and the right exercise plan reported an enhanced quality of life! Exercising regularly has been known to improve bone health and reduce the loss of bone density by conserving bone tissue, especially for females in their post-menopausal phase.

People with osteoporosis are generally known to have poor posture, feeble bones, and weak muscles that lead to frequent falls and fall-associated fractures. Adopting the right exercise plan improves muscle strength and promotes balance in people with osteoporosis. With the right amount of balance and muscle-strengthening activities, your risk of falling can be lessened. Weight-bearing exercises, resistance training, and flexibility exercises have been proven to prevent bone loss, mitigate pain, and promote overall health. It is never too late to start exercising! Exercise is important to keep yourself active and healthy and prevent frequent falls associated with osteoporosis. A detailed guideline on the right exercises (and how to do them) is provided in chapters 4 and 5 as part of your new comprehensive osteoporosis health plan

Chapter 2

The Diet Connection

A well-balanced diet is crucial to improving the conditions associated with osteoporosis. In fact, dietary habits are even known to enhance bone health. A healthy, balanced diet strengthens the bones, muscles, and joints and certain nutrients such as calcium, magnesium, and vitamin D play an important role in both the development and prevention of osteoporosis.

The Link Between Food And Bone Health

It's true that what you eat determines your overall health. Nutrients (which are a modifiable risk factor) that are present in food are known to impact bone health. The food we eat can alter the entire structure of our bones and even the rate at which our body heals itself. Generally speaking, the prevention of osteoporosis and other related bone disorders begins during early childhood, when the intake of a calcium-rich diet is essential in order to promote the long-term health and formation of bones. A well-balanced diet rich in essential bone nutrients (which we'll cover later in this chapter) enhances the process of bone formation while preventing bone loss.

There are various dietary components, such as micro and macronutrients, which enhance bone health and assist in the quick healing of fractured bones. On the other hand, deficiencies in major essential nutrients (such as vitamins and calcium) slow down or completely diminish the healing process in bones. A trademark of osteoporosis is the associated fragility fractures that occur due to poor bone health. Alcoholic drinks, caffeine, and certain food products, such as high-salt foods, may damage and weaken the bones, resulting in brittleness and fractures.

Micronutrients And Osteoporosis

One of the primary groups of nutrients required by your body is called "micronutrients." Carbohydrates, fats, and proteins are classified as macronutrients, whereas most vitamins and minerals are classified as micronutrients. Adequate quantities of micronutrients are essential for maintaining optimal health and preventing diseases, and, as the name suggests, they are only required in small quantities. It is important to note that, although only small amounts are required, deficiencies in micronutrients can result in several devastating and severe consequences.

In addition, to maintain optimal health, micronutrients play an important role in promoting and maintaining the bone health of an individual. With the exception of vitamin D, micronutrients are not produced naturally in the body. Therefore, it is essential that we obtain the required quantities of micronutrients through the food that we eat.

Calcium and Vitamin D are the two most essential micronutrients required for the prevention of bone loss and they work hand in hand. Calcium is an essential mineral nutrient for bone development as well as a significant component in combating osteoporosis, and our bones hold a major reservoir of calcium for our bodies. When a sufficient quantity of calcium is not obtained from one's diet, the body pulls calcium from the bones, thereby making the bones weak and susceptible to fractures. Consuming a sufficient amount of calcium makes our bones strong while vitamin D helps the body absorb the calcium, which prevents further bone loss (especially for those with osteoporosis.) Additionally, there are various other micronutrients that are important for optimal bone health. For example, magnesium increases bone density and vitamin K helps bind calcium and other essential minerals to the bone, making our bones stronger and helping to prevent fractures.

According to a study done by Genius and Bouchard (2012) on the Combination of Micronutrients for Bone (COMB), it is observed that, along with daily exercise, a micronutrient combination regimen (which included vitamins such as vitamin D3 and K2 and minerals such as strontium, magnesium, and docosahexaenoic acid (DHA)) was found to be more effective for increasing bone density in osteoporosis patients than simply using bisphosphonate drug therapy.

A lifestyle that incorporates a healthy diet plan and regular exercise is known to enhance strong and healthy bones. The key nutrients that promote bone health and require considerate attention include calcium, vitamin D, protein, vitamin C, magnesium, vitamin K, and zinc. It is important to include these nutrients in your daily meal plan to boost the health of your bones.

Calcium is required for building strong bones and is abundantly found in dairy products. The daily Recommended Dietary Allowance (RDA) of calcium varies according to your age group.

Table 2.1: Recommended Calcium Intake for Different Age Groups

Age Group (years)	Recommended Dietary Allowance (RDA)	
	Male (mg/day)	Female (mg/day)
2-11	1000	1000
11-19	1300	1300
19-50	1000	1000
50-70	1000	1200
Above 70	1200	1200

Vitamin D is responsible for calcium absorption and can often be found in fish and eggs. The RDA of vitamin D intake is as follows:

Table 2.2: Recommended Vitamin D Intake for
Different Age Groups

Age Group (years)	Recommended Dietary Allowance (RDA)	
	Male (mcg/day)	Female(mcg/day)
2-13	15	15
14-19	15	15
19-50	15	15
50-70	15	15
Above 70	20	20

Protein makes up to 50 percent of one's bone volume. Food sources such as beans, legumes, and salmon are rich in protein. T. Beans are an excellent source of calcium, magnesium, fiber, and other essential nutrients. However, they also contain phytates, which can impede your body's ability to absorb the calcium present in them. To effectively reduce phytate levels, simply soak the beans in water for several hours and then cook them in fresh water. This method enhances nutrient absorption, allowing you to benefit from the nutritional value of beans fully.he RDA of protein is as follows:

Table 2.3: Recommended Protein Intake for Different Age Groups

Age Group (years)	Recommended Dietary Allowance (RDA)	
	Male (grams/kg/day)	Female(grams/kg/day)
3-15	0.9	0.9
15-19	0.9	0.8
19-50	0.8	0.8
50-70	1-1.2	1-1.2

Above 70	1-1.2	1-1.2

Vitamin C is known to prevent bone loss and maintain the health of bones. The RDA of vitamin C is as follows:

Table 2.4: Recommended Vitamin C Intake for Different Age Groups

Age Group (years)	Recommended Dietary Allowance (RDA)	
	Male (mg/day)	Female(mg/day)
9-15	45	45
15-19	65	65
19-50	90	75
50-70	75	75
Above 70	75	75

Magnesium plays a major role in preventing the risk of bone fractures by increasing bone density and maintaining bone health. The RDA of magnesium is as follows:

Table 2.5: Recommended Magnesium Intake for Different Age Groups

Age Group (years)	Recommended Dietary Allowance (RDA)	
	Male (mg/day)	Female(mg/day)
9-13	240	240
14-18	410	360
19-30	400	310
31-50	420	320
Above 50	420	320

Vitamin K plays a vital role in building bone mineral density and is involved in reducing the risk of bone fractures. The RDA of vitamin K is as follows:

Table 2.6: Recommended Vitamin K Intake for Different Age Groups

Age Group (years)	Recommended Dietary Allowance (RDA)	
	Male (mcg/day)	Female(mcg/day)
9-13	60	60
14-18	75	75
19-30	120	90
31-50	120	90
Above 50	120	90

Zinc plays an important role in healing bones. Shellfish, legumes, and meat are some of the primary sources of dietary zinc. The RDA of zinc is as follows:

Table 2.7: Recommended Zinc Intake for Different Age Groups

Age Group (years)	Recommended Dietary Allowance (RDA)	
	Male (mg/day)	Female(mg/day)
9-13	8	8
14-18	11	9
19-30	11	8
31-50	11	8
Above 50	9.4	6.8

Diet For Good Bone Health

Along with regular exercise, good bone health is enhanced by the intake of a well-balanced diet that includes all the nutrients required for promoting bone health. Consuming a diet with a good nutrient composition instead of a diet with high amounts of fat, salt, and sugar is required to maintain bone health. The safest strategy is to consume a low-salt diet that includes plenty of fresh and minimally processed whole grains, fruits, and vegetables.

Additionally, choosing fat-free and low-fat calcium-rich dairy products and foods rich in vitamin D will contribute greatly to a bone-healthy diet. This diet should include plenty of vegetables such as beets, turnips, broccoli, tomatoes, cabbage, parsley, potatoes, red and green peppers, kale, and okra. It is also important to include dairy products, sardines and/or salmon, meat (and other high-protein foods), legumes, and fruits such as grapefruit, strawberries, pineapple, avocados, papayas, oranges, lemons, mangoes, and prunes.

Including foods that are rich in calcium and vitamin D promotes the overall health of bones.

Similarly, certain food products interfere with bone health. Since foods that contain high quantities of salt are known to cause bone loss, it is essential to limit one's intake of salty foods. Many canned and processed foods have a high salt content; therefore, it is important to limit the intake of these foods to maintain bone strength. Similarly, caffeinated drinks such as coffee, tea, and certain carbonated soft drinks interfere with the calcium absorption in the body which, in turn, leads to bone loss.

In addition to causing various other health issues, both smoking and alcohol intake are known to have a negative impact on bone health and hence should be avoided. Smoking alters the ability of the body to absorb calcium which, in turn, leads to lower bone density and fractured bones. Similarly, excessive alcohol intake increases the risk of osteoporosis by affecting the bone density and mechanical properties of the bones. Chronic alcohol consumption decreases the process of bone formation and increases the rate of bone deterioration. So, I strongly urge you to stay away from both smoking and excessive alcohol intake as a part of maintaining your bone health.

Food Groups That Fight Bone Loss And Rebuild Bones

I know it can sound like there is a lot to consider when it comes to building a good diet for preserving and repairing bone health. But it is absolutely possible to easily include the essential micronutrients that your bones need through food that is both enjoyable as well as accessible. Just remember to consume these highly recommended food groups that are rich in bone nutrients to combat osteoporosis. They include dairy products, nuts, fruits and vegetables, and fatty fish.

Dairy products that are rich in calcium (such as cheese, milk, butter, and yogurt) are found to increase bone growth in children, improve bone density in adolescents, and diminish the rate of bone deterioration in adults. For older adults, calcium-rich dairy products are known to improve bone density and reduce the risk of falls and fall-related fractures. An intake of two to three servings of milk per day provides an adequate amount of calcium required for the growth and strengthening of bones. Calcium-rich products are also involved in the healing of bone fractures. Apart from being rich in calcium, dairy products that fortify the bone are also known to contain various other bone nutrients such as protein, phosphorous, and vitamin K2.

Nuts are another important food group that should be included in any diet with the goal of strengthening one's bone health. Nuts such as almonds, walnuts, pecans, and peanuts contain essential bone nutrients such as calcium, magnesium, and phosphorous. Consuming a handful of almonds each day is known to effectively boost the levels of magnesium and phosphorous – nutrients that are required for the growth and development of bones.

Green vegetables that include cabbage, kale, collard greens, turnip greens, broccoli, beans, and mustard greens are found to be rich in calcium. Similarly, plantains, sweet potatoes, and raisins are rich in magnesium. Intake of papaya, orange, and prunes that are rich in potassium and grapefruits, strawberries, and pineapples rich in pineapples strongly enhances the growth and repair of bones. Canned sardines and salmon fishes that are rich in calcium and fatty fish like salmon, mackerel, tuna, and sardines that are rich in Vitamin D promote bone health by preventing bone loss.

Well-cooked turnip greens, consuming a baked potato without adding salt, adding grapefruit to breakfast, intake of fresh dried figs, canned salmons, sandwiches with almond butter spread, and fortified orange juice are some of the rewarding food that boosts bone health.

Dietary Guidelines To Manage Osteoporosis

In addition to performing regular exercise, consuming adequate quantities of essential key nutrients helps to manage osteoporosis. Dairy products, nuts, fruits and vegetables, and fatty fish that are rich in these micronutrients are involved in the bone remodeling process and are highly recommended by the NOF. They're even considered an essential food group for reducing inflammation and other stress-related disorders in osteoporosis patients. For elderly people, a bone-healthy diet can even slow down the process of bone loss and stabilize bone health, thereby reducing the risk of falls and fall-related fractures. To prevent and treat osteoporosis, NOF recommends the intake of sufficient amounts of the required bone nutrients from quality food sources such as low-fat milk, cheese, yogurt, sardines, salmon, tuna, okra, turnips, cabbage, broccoli, tomatoes, raisins, potatoes, pineapple, and leafy vegetables. Soy products such as tofu, soy beverages, and tempeh are actually **beneficial for bone health**.

They are rich in calcium and protein and contain compounds called isoflavones that help reduce bone breakdown. Including these foods in your diet can help maintain bone strength and reduce the risk of osteoporosis.

Some notable dietary guidelines include:

i.   adopting a well-balanced nutritious diet

ii.   increasing fruit and vegetable intake

iii.   reducing sodium

iv.   intake consuming only a moderate amount of caffeinated drinks

v.   restricting alcohol intake

Consuming the recommended daily amount of key bone nutrients found in these foods helps in attaining bone health by preventing further bone loss in older adults.

When the recommended quantities of the dietary essential nutrients are unavailable to the body, it must be compensated through the intake of supplements. Even though the intake of dietary vitamin A through yellow and orange vegetables contributes significantly to increasing one's bone strength, an excessive intake (or even a slight increase) of vitamin A through substances such as liver or cod liver oil is considered harmful to bones. Too much vitamin A can actually decrease bone density and increase the rate of hip fractures! So, I highly recommend you consult your doctor before starting a new supplement routine.

Food Groups To Approach With Caution

Although many foods alleviate osteoporosis symptoms, there are certain foods that I recommend you avoid or approach with caution due to their potential negative effects on bone health. These include salt, soft drinks, and caffeine. These foods inhibit the body from absorbing calcium and diminish the BMD.

Out of the many diet dangers for osteoporosis patients, reducing the intake of salt is often the most challenging. Salt poses a major threat to the skeletal bones and is linked with faster bone loss, especially for postmenopausal women. In fact, postmenopausal women who consume a high-salt diet often experience faster bone loss than postmenopausal women of the same age who consume a low-salt diet.

The overabundance of table salt in the typical American diet is one of the causes of such high calcium requirements in the body. Cooking with too much salt and eating processed foods such as hot dogs, ham, fast food, pizza, and burgers can easily add too much sodium to your diet. Most canned foods such as soups, vegetables, juices, and certain baked products are high in salt content. Hence, it is better to avoid these foods for maintaining optimal bone health, especially for elderly people and for those diagnosed with osteoporosis.

Luckily, the recommended quantity of calcium and vitamin D can compensate for the bone loss brought on by excessive salt intake in osteoporosis patients. Additionally, consuming high amounts of potassium-rich foods such as tomatoes, orange juice, and bananas helps reduce the calcium loss in bones caused by the intake of foods with a high salt content.

Most sodas and carbonated soft drinks are rich in phosphoric acid, which also contributes to an abundant loss of calcium in the body. Therefore, limiting the intake of these kinds of carbonated drinks enhances the health of bones, especially for people with osteoporosis. In limited quantities, soda that is free of phosphoric acid can be used as a replacement for drinks with phosphoric acid.

Caffeinated products are also important for osteoporosis patients to avoid. This is because caffeine intake drains calcium from the bones. Since coffee is a rich source of caffeine, I would strongly suggest you restrict the intake of coffee to prevent further bone loss.

A Bone Health Diet Food List

FOOD	Examples	NUTRIENTS
Dairy products	Low-fat milk, yogurt, cheese	Calcium, Vitamin D
Nuts	Pistachios, Almonds, Sunflower seeds	Calcium, Magnesium
Fishes	Canned Sardines, Salmon	Calcium
	Salmon, Mackerel, Tuna	Vitamin D

Fruits & Vegetables	Kale, Okra, Cabbage, Broccoli	Calcium
	Beet greens, Potatoes, Plantains, Tomatoes	Magnesium
	Papayas, Oranges, Bananas, Prunes	Potassium
	Red & Green Peppers, Grapefruit	Vitamin C
	Dark green leafy vegetables	Vitamin K

Others	Cereals, Snacks, Bread	Calcium, vitamin D
	Meat, Shellfish, Poultry	Zinc
	Eggs	Protein, Vitamin D

Chapter 3

Before You Get Moving

This chapter focuses on the safety aspects that must be considered as part of a comprehensive plan for improving the health of your bones. All the exercises described here have clinically proven successful and are considered safe for people with osteoporosis to perform at home. Through clinical assessments, you and your doctor/physical therapist can work together to choose the most suitable exercises for you.

Stick With The Right Flexibility Level

Exercising regularly can greatly reduce the loss of bone density associated with osteoporosis. Regular exercise, which is regarded as an important care component in managing osteoporosis, helps to improve bone strength and balance for osteoporosis patients.

However, not all exercises will be beneficial. Therefore, it is essential to choose correct, effective, and safe exercises to help improve your body's overall flexibility. Pain is a normal indicator that the body exhibits while performing exercises but carrying out workouts that are too strenuous ends up causing more damage to bones than benefits.

While working to improve bone health, it is important to start with low-level, light-weight exercises with few repetitions before slowly progressing to the next level. Performing vigorous exercises too quickly is known to increase the risk of falls and fall-related injuries.

Benefits Of Simple Stretches

Stretching is an important physical activity that improves overall health and should be incorporated into the daily routine of any person, with or without osteoporosis.

For those with osteoporosis, it is found that simple stretching increases flexibility, the prime factor of bone fitness. Stretching warms and relaxes the muscles and joints and is known to improve posture and reduce the physical and mental stress in people with osteoporosis. It also helps to diminish the pain associated with muscle tightness.

Aside from these advantages, stretching is also beneficial for increasing the range of motion, enhancing the performance of physical activities, encouraging blood flow to the muscles, promoting quick healing, and preventing back pain.

Stretching includes various techniques such as dynamic, static, ballistic, and active stretching. Of these, the dynamic and the static forms are the most common types of stretching. We will learn more about the various types of stretches you can do in Chapter 4.

According to the NIH Osteoporosis and Related Bone Diseases National Resource Center, regular exercise plays a crucial role in healing people with osteoporosis. Carrying out the stretching activities recommended by your health care provider for at least 5-10 minutes after each osteoporosis workout has been found to improve the bone health of people with osteoporosis.

Exercises To Avoid

Even though performing exercises has been found to be of great advantage in promoting bone health for people with osteoporosis, according to the NOF, there are certain types of exercises that people with low bone density must avoid. This is because certain activities and movements can increase the risk of hip, spine, and wrist fractures and end up worsening your health condition rather than enhancing your overall wellness. The exercises that need to be avoided include high-impact exercises such as running, jumping, bending, twisting, sit-ups, and toe touches. Both high-impact and excessive bending and twisting exercises have been found to trigger a series of fractures in people with poor bone health. Therefore, these kinds of exercises should be avoided.

Furthermore, certain yoga and Pilates poses such as rounded spine movements, spine twists, and deep hip stretches present a high risk for spine fractures. For similar reasons, golf, tennis, skiing, and other high-fall-risk sports should also be avoided for people with poor bone health.

Determining Your Fracture Risk Level

We've learned that exercise stimulates bone health by preventing further bone loss and decreasing the risk of falls and fall-related fractures, but what is the best way to get started with a new exercise plan? Assessing and identifying your risk for bone fractures is the first step to take to start the best osteoporosis exercise plan for you.

There are several ways to assess the risk for fractures in an individual, such as assessment tools and bone scans. Even though these fracture risk assessment measures are generally recommended by a doctor, there are currently various online assessment tools to identify your current and future fracture risk levels. The online tool uses a questionnaire to gather information such as your age, health condition, gender, family history, medications, and history of previous falls and then calculates your risk for fragility factors for the next ten years. These online assessment tools are designed to assess and predict risk levels for individuals in certain age groups and may or may not be a good fit for you.

One common online tool that is widely accepted for assessing the risk for bone fractures is called the 'Ten-year Fracture Risk Calculator,' designed by American Bone Health. This tool estimates the risk of bone fractures for men and women who are over the age of 45. If the results obtained from the assessment tool indicate that one's risk level is close to the point of requiring treatment, then bone scans are recommended for further assessment. Bone scans measure bone density and are the most widely used measure for diagnosing osteoporosis.

Setting And Maintaining A Routine

Performing exercises regularly maintains bone mass and reduces the risk of falls and fall-related fractures and is an essential component of every osteoporosis management regimen. In order to stay motivated and committed to performing our exercises regularly, it is good to start slow and progress intentionally over time toward the goal of improving both our bone health as well as our overall health. It is essential to listen to your body before continuing with an exercise plan. It is normal to experience muscle pain and/or soreness but pain that lasts for more than 48 hours indicates that the workouts carried out were too strenuous! Remember, a slow and steady pace is key.

In order to promote bone health, the NIH recommends carrying out exercises daily for at least 30 minutes. When it comes to setting and sticking with an exercise regimen, it helps to start with a clear goal in mind. For some people, the goal is to improve bone density. For others, it's to prevent falls and fall-related fractures.

Your exercise routine plan should be designed based on your age, severity of osteoporosis, current medications, fitness level, and other medical conditions. For those with osteoporosis, a plan that includes a combination of weight-bearing aerobic exercises, resistance exercises, stretching, and balance exercises has proven to be useful for promoting bone health and improving quality of life. Hence, those with osteoporosis need to stick with a customized exercise plan with sincerity and commitment.

Ready To Start?

It is of utmost importance for people with osteoporosis to perform physical activities with appropriate safety and caution. Exercises to manage osteoporosis should be done regularly and for the proper length of time. Before each exercise session, a gentle warm-up routine is required to introduce your body to that portion of your osteoporosis exercise plan. Warming up helps boost blood circulation and prepares the joints and muscles for exercise. Exercises should be done slowly with a gradual warm-up consisting of gentle stretches.

It is best for people with osteoporosis to start their exercise plan with low-impact physical activities and steadily increase to high-impact exercises over time. Carry out every activity slowly. Perform 8-10 repetitions, being sure to rest for 10-15 seconds after each repetition. For weight-bearing exercises, be careful not to increase the weight too much or too soon! Instead, weight should be increased gradually to improve the strength and health of your bones.

It is important to take your current health condition and other factors into consideration before carrying out any physical activities. If you experience any sort of discomfort or pain while performing exercises, immediately stop the exercise plan and consult a doctor before proceeding with further exercise.

Equipment Needs

Since the exercises described in this osteoporosis exercise plan can be performed at home, the equipment required for this regimen is mostly available at home.

Common pieces of equipment that may be required include a sturdy chair with a high back and no arms, a jump rope, dumbbells, ankle weights, a non-slip mat, loop bands, foam rollers, straps, or an old belt (for stretching activities), and a pair of wrist weights.

There are also other budget-friendly and easily available objects and equipment that may be required for your exercise routine, including a therapy ball, free weights, and elastic exercise bands. Other optional equipment may include an elliptical machine, a vibration platform, or a functional trainer where multiple strengthening exercises may be performed.

Chapter 4

24 Moves To Stop Bone Loss And Rebuild Bones

With the following exercises, you can reduce bone loss and rebuild skeletal bones. This chapter focuses on the most effective at-home exercises that you can do to combat osteoporosis and its related fractures. The exercises highlighted in this chapter are good options to help strengthen your bones, prevent bone loss, promote good posture, and improve balance.

Strength Training Exercises

Exercises to Prevent Bone Loss and Build Strong Bones

Resistance exercises are crucial components in developing stronger bones. These exercises make the muscles in your arms, legs, and spine work harder and, over time, become stronger. Strong spinal muscles are imperative for having good posture. Resistance training also adds the right amount of stress on bones necessary to help improve bone density.

Movement: **Standing Partial Squats**

Flexibility level: **Beginner**

***Description*:**

- Stand on a firm surface with feet shoulder-width apart
- Tighten your tummy muscles to engage your core
- Gently squat down halfway (you should feel the muscles in your thighs and butt tightening)

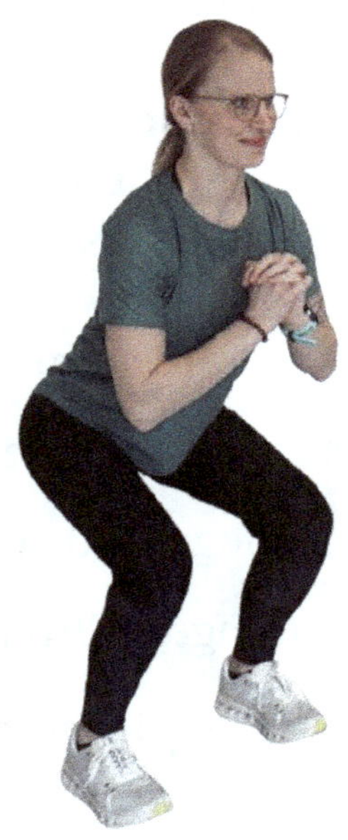

- Hold this position for 1-2 seconds and stand back up

What this does: The muscles in your hip and knee will contract, which will aid in strengthening and supporting your bones. This movement will also help load your hip and knee bones which will help improve bone density.

Repetition: Repeat this movement 7-10 times per set, once a day. Perform 3 sets. Try starting with 7 reps and gradually progressing to 10 reps.

Good for: Improving your standing tolerance for brushing your teeth, cooking, and performing other chores that require prolonged standing. These exercises will also be beneficial for activities such as mowing your lawn or bird watching.

Movement: **Bicep Curls**

Flexibility: **Beginner**

Description:

- Sit on a firm surface with feet shoulder-width apart
- Hold 1–2-pound dumbbells in each hand, palms up, in front of your body, and bend your elbows towards your chest (you should feel your muscles tightening in your arms)
- Hold this for 1-2 seconds, then straighten your elbows

What this does: The muscles in your hands, elbows, forearms, and arms will contract, which will help strengthen and support your bones. The weight in your hands will help improve the weight-bearing capability in your hands, elbows, and shoulders, which in turn helps with increasing bone density.

Repetition: Repeat this movement 7-10 times per set, once a day. Perform 3 sets. Try starting with 7 reps and slowly progressing to 10 reps.

Good for: Increasing your ability to carry groceries, pull a door open, and perform other repeated activities.

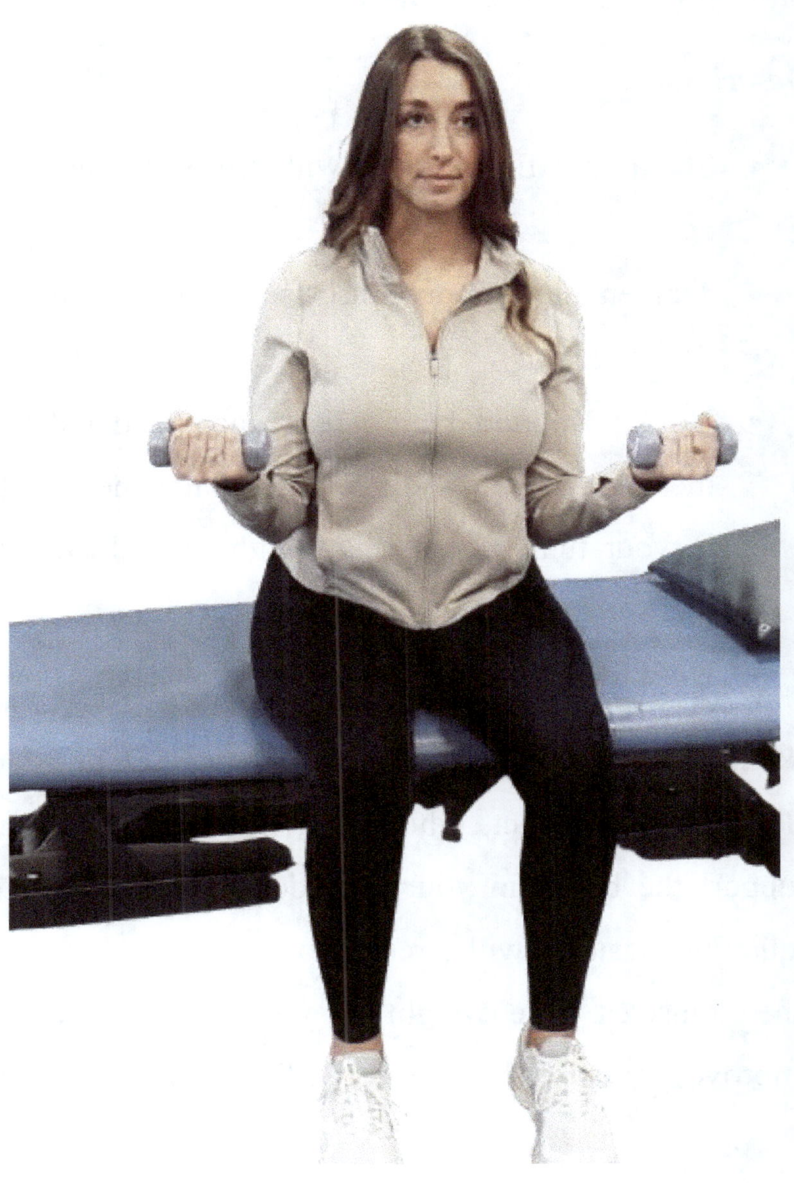

Movement: **Partial Squat Position Shoulder Press with Dumbbells**

Flexibility level: **Intermediate**

***Description*:**

- Stand on a firm surface with feet shoulder-width apart
- Tighten your tummy muscles to engage your core
- Squat partially
- Hold 2-3-pound dumbbells in each hand and raise them above your head (you should feel the muscles in your tummy, buttocks, thighs, shoulders, and elbows tightening)
- Hold for 1-2 seconds and lower the weights down.

What this does: The muscles in your shoulders and elbows will contract, which will help strengthen and support the bones in your shoulders and elbows. The squatting position will strengthen your core, hips, and knee muscles. The weight in your hands will help improve your weight-bearing ability in your humerus (the main bone in your arm) and thoracic spine (upper back) which, in turn, helps with increasing bone density.

Repetition: Repeat this movement 7-10 times per set, once a day. Perform 3 sets. Try starting with 7 reps and progressing to 10 reps.

Good for: Improving your ability to reach overhead and lift above your shoulder level. This will help you with gardening, vacuuming, and other similar activities.

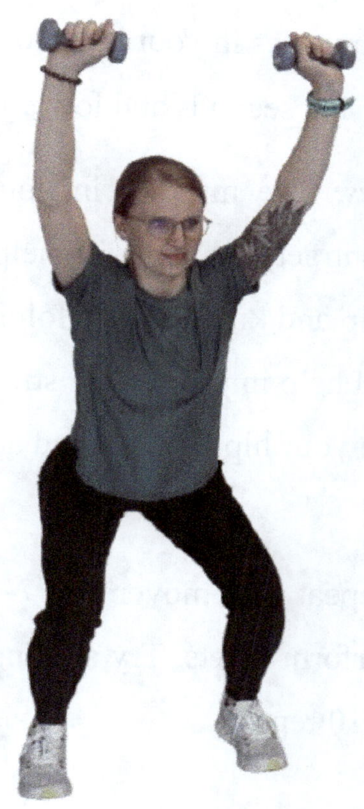

Movement: **Partial Squats with Ball Behind Back**

Flexibility level: **Intermediate**

Description:

- Stand on a firm surface with feet shoulder-width apart, close to a wall
- Hold a 2-3-pound dumbbell in each hand
- Place a gym ball behind your lower back
- Gently squat down to your knee level (you should feel the muscles in your hip and thighs tightening)
- Hold for 1-2 seconds and lower the weights down

What this does: The muscles in your hips, butt, and thighs will contract, which will help strengthen and support your hip and knee bones. Holding the weights in your hands will help improve your strength and increase bone density in your hips, knees, and ankles, stimulating bone growth.

Repetition: Repeat this movement 7-10 times per set, once a day. Perform 3 sets. Try starting with 7 reps and progressing to 10 reps.

Good for: Improving your ability to walk for long distances and to perform activities such as standing and pulling your pants up. It may also improve your balance for activities that require standing.

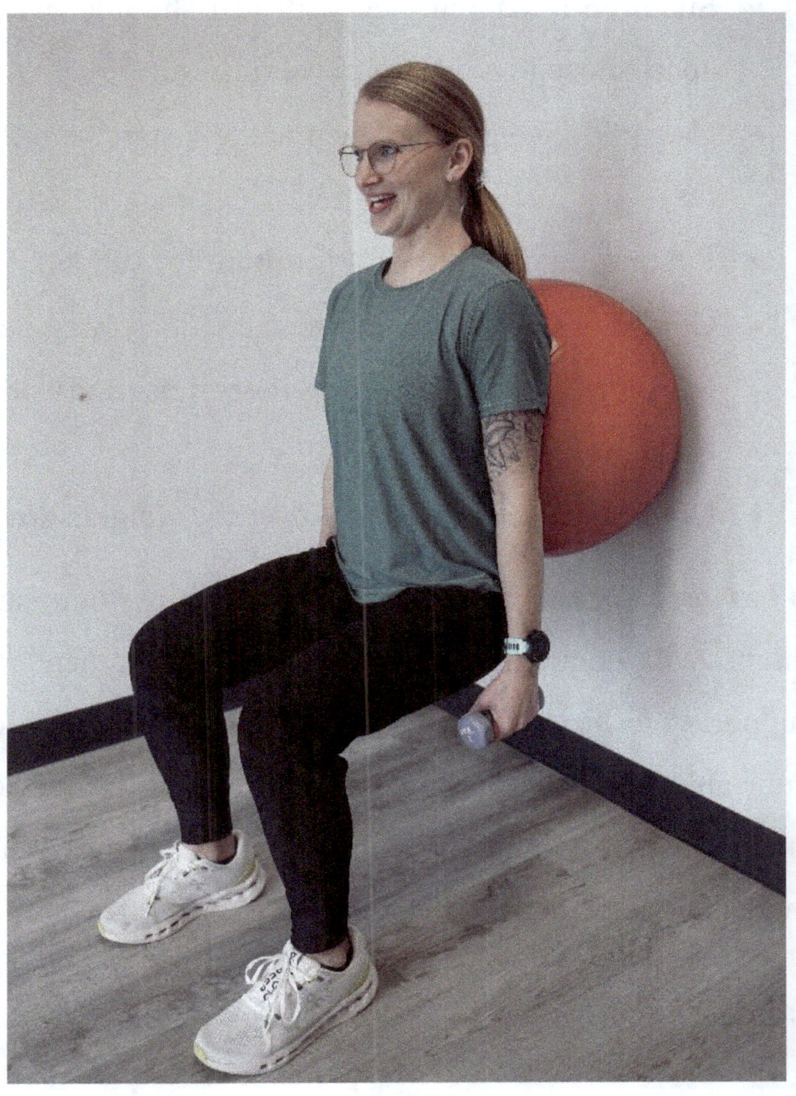

Movement: **Sideways Leg Lift**

Flexibility level: **Advanced**

Description:

- Stand on a firm surface with feet shoulder-width apart, close to a wall or piece of furniture
- Use ankle weights on each ankle (start with 2-3 lbs)
- Put one hand on the wall/furniture for support
- Gently bring one leg out to the side (you should feel the muscles behind your hips and sides tightening)
- Hold for 1-2 seconds and lower the weights down

What this does: The muscles in your hips, butt, and thighs will contract, which will help strengthen and support your hip and knee bones. Lifting the weights on your ankles will help improve your strength in that leg and bearing weight on your other leg helps with increasing bone density by stimulating bone growth.

Repetition: Alternate sides. Repeat this movement 7-10 times per set, once a day. Perform 3 sets. Try starting with 7 reps and progressing to 10 reps.

Good for: Improving your stability, balance, and ability to walk outdoors on grass and get out of your chair and car.

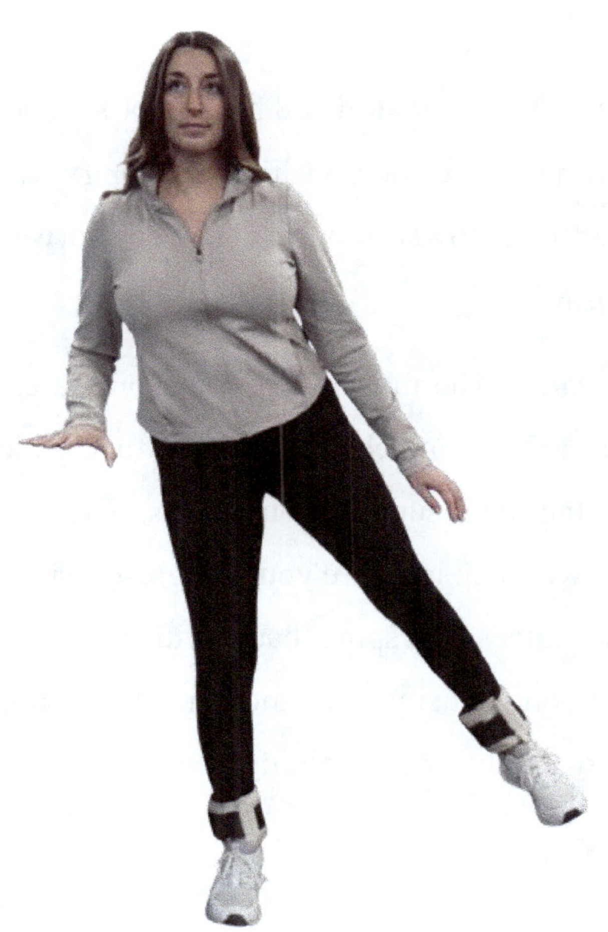

Movement: **Forward Lunges with Weight**

Flexibility level: **Advanced**

Description:

- Stand with one foot forward while holding a 2-3-pound dumbbell in each hand
- Engage your core muscles by tucking your tummy in.
- Gently lunge forward and hold for 1 second.
- Return to a standing position and lunge with your other foot, slowly moving your body forward
- Repeat

What this does: The muscles in your spine area, core, hips, knees, ankles, and elbows will contract, which will help strengthen and support your bones. The weight in your hands will help improve your weight-bearing ability in your hips, knees, and spine (back) which, in turn, helps to increase bone density. This movement also improves balance and stability with walking.

Repetition: Repeat this movement 10 times per set, once a day. Perform 3-4 sets. Try starting with 7 reps and progressing to 10 reps per set.

Good for: Improving overall balance and your ability to walk, climb stairs, kneel, squat for gardening, and tolerate standing activities at home.

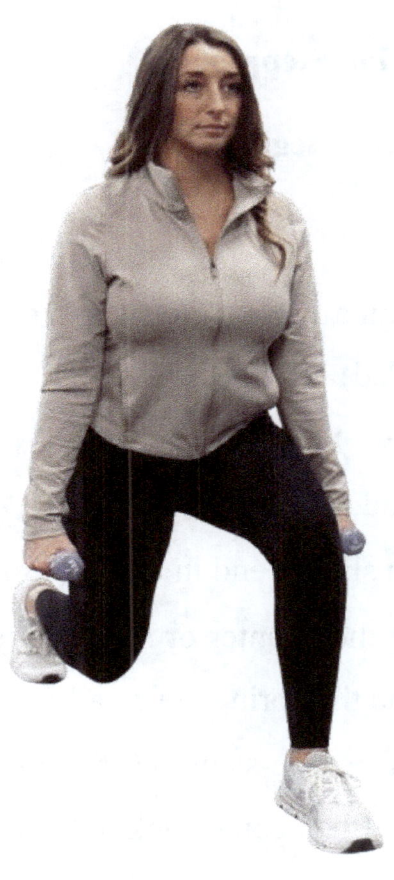

Weight Bearing Exercises

Weight-bearing exercises play a major role in improving bone density. These are exercises you do on your feet – making your bones and muscles work against gravity to keep you in an upright position. Low-impact weight-bearing exercises such as walking reinforce and reduce bone loss in your legs and lumbar spine.

Movement: **Side Stepping**

Flexibility level: **Beginner**

Description:

- Stand on a firm surface near a counter (for support if needed)
- Tighten your tummy muscles to engage your core/abdomen
- Keep a slight bend in both of your knees
- Facing the counter or support surface, step to the side and then bring your trailing foot back together
- Continue side-stepping for the length of your counter, then come back in the other direction.

- Tip: Use the counter or surface for support as needed. If your balance is good and you feel steady, try completing these exercises without using the support surface.

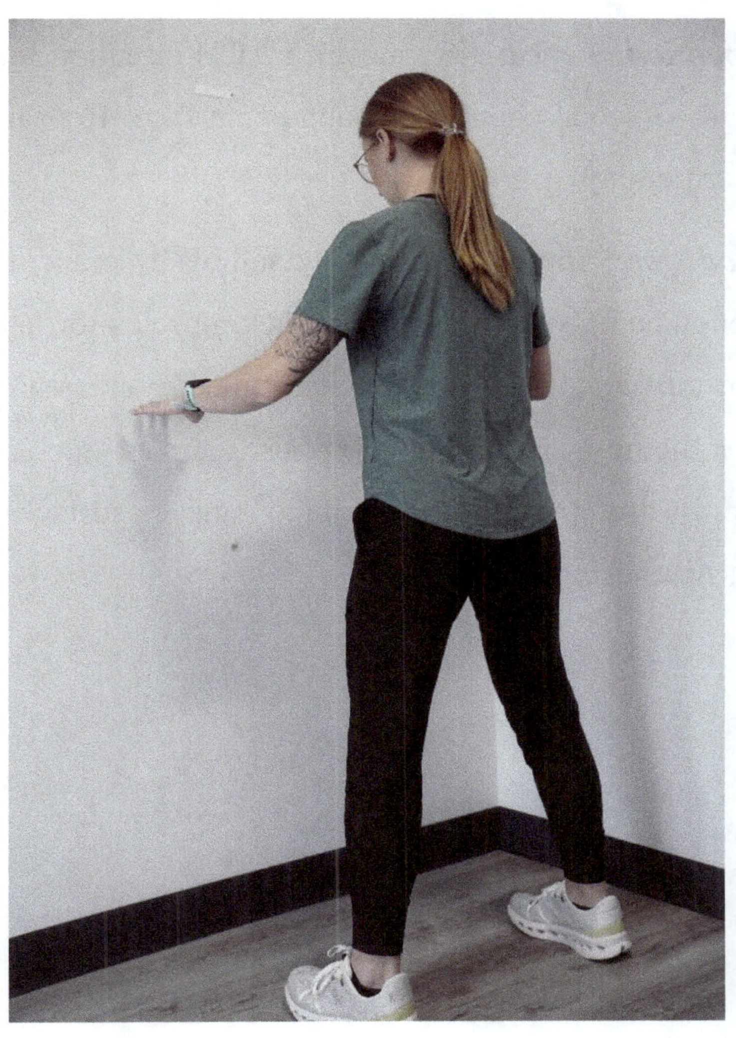

What this does: The muscles in your side hip area will be activated, which aids in balance and stability for walking and climbing stairs. Your core/abdomen will also be engaged throughout, furthering your stability and balance.

Repetition: Repeat 3-5 times in EACH direction for the length of your counter or support surface. Repeat 1-2 times per day.

Good for: Improving your standing tolerance and strengthening your hips and buttock muscles for lateral-type movements in your kitchen or other areas around your home. These exercises also aid in increasing stability and strength for walking on uneven surfaces like grass and using stairs.

Movement: **Wall Push-Ups**

Flexibility level: **Beginner**

Description:

- Stand on a firm surface about 2 feet away from the wall

- Place hands on wall (about shoulder height and slightly farther than shoulder-width apart)

- Start with arms extended, then slowly bend elbows, bringing your body closer to the wall

- Keep your feet flat on the floor, engaging your tummy muscles

- Keep your back straight (as if there were a board on your back)

- Straighten your arms back out to return to the starting position

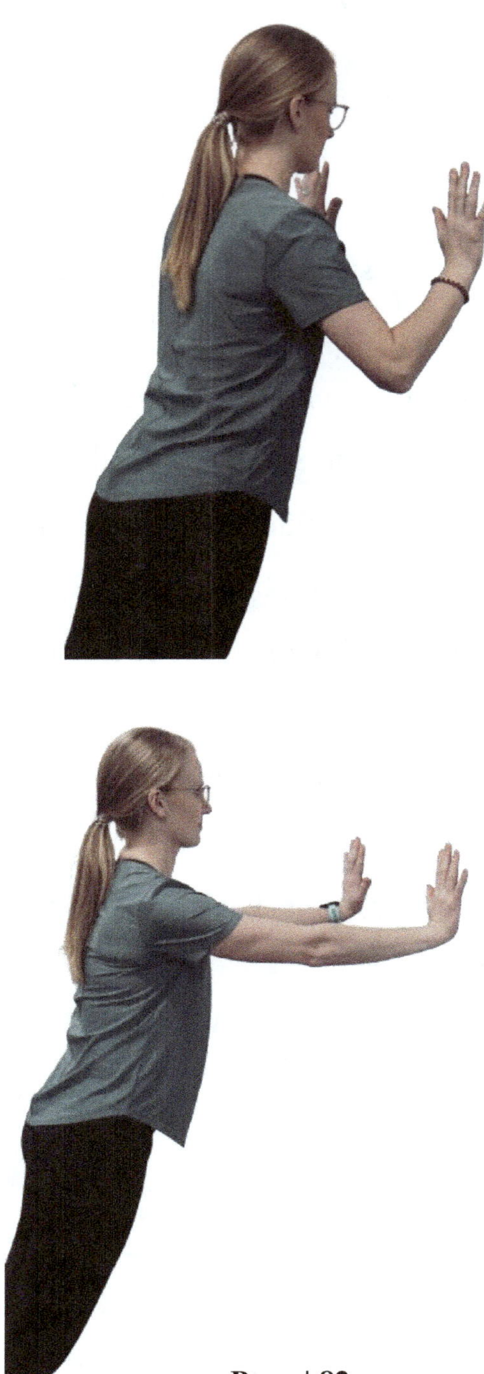

What this does: Strengthens your shoulder and chest muscles while keeping your tummy muscles engaged. This helps increase stability and balance for daily tasks while protecting your lower back.

Repetition: Perform 7-10 reps per set, once per day—complete 3 sets total. Try starting with 7 reps and progressing to 10 reps as you feel able and comfortable. Discontinue if you experience any pain.

Good for: Strengthening your shoulder and chest muscles, which will aid in your ability to lift various items into your cupboard, wash/comb your hair, and push/pull open doors.

Movement: **Forward and Lateral Step-Ups**

Flexibility level: **Intermediate**

Description:

- Stand at the bottom of a step, holding onto railings for support as needed
- Tighten your tummy muscles to engage your core
- Starting with your right foot, step up onto the bottom step (one foot at a time – both feet will end up on the bottom step)
- Starting with your right foot, return each foot to the floor
- Repeat the same process, starting with your left foot. Hold onto a railing for support as needed
- Stand facing the railing and repeat the exercises, moving side to side instead of forward/backward.

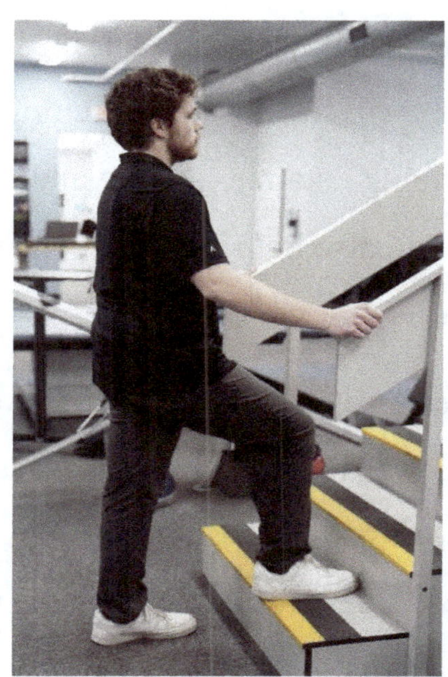

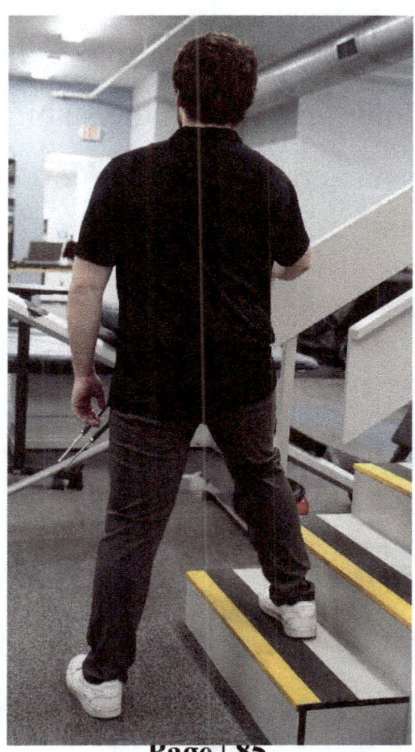

What this does: The muscles in your hips and thighs will contract, which will aid in strengthening your legs for walking, climbing stairs, and walking on uneven surfaces. This will also help increase bone density in your hips and lower legs.

Repetition: Perform 7-10 reps, leading with each foot, going both forward and sideways up and down the bottom step. Start with 7 reps for each leg, building up to 10 reps on each side. Hold onto stair railings as needed for support and safety.

Good for: Strengthening your hips, glutes, and thigh muscles and aiding in building the stability necessary to negotiate stairs and curbs in the community.

Movement: **Table Level Plank**

Flexibility level: **Intermediate**

Description:

- Stand on a firm, non-slippery surface with hands on a tabletop
- Tighten your tummy muscles to engage your core
- Slowly walk your feet backward, away from the table, until you're in a plank position
- Hold that position for 10-30 seconds, maintaining a straight spine, your head and neck in a neutral position
- Stop immediately if you experience an onset of pain.

What this does: Engages core/abdominal muscles to increase stability required for various types of activities of daily living.

Repetition: Perform 3 times, holding for 10-30 seconds each time. Begin with 10 seconds, and then build up to 30 seconds.

Good for: Increasing core strength and stability for standing activities like cooking, cleaning, dressing, and various other activities of daily living.

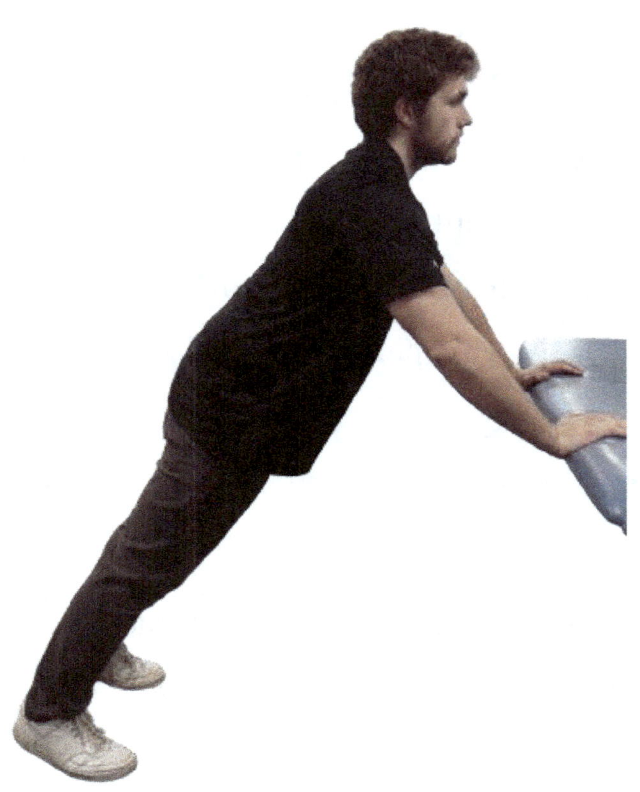

Movement: **Calf/Heel Raises**

Flexibility level: **Advanced**

Description:

- Stand on a firm surface near a counter (for stability and safety as needed), with your feet flat on the floor
- Push through your toes, raising your heels off the floor as high as possible

- Hold for 1-2 seconds, then lower back to starting position

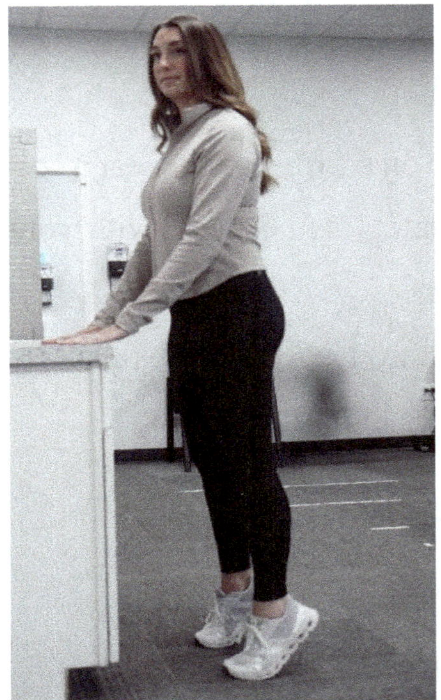

What this does: Activates your lower leg muscles for foot/ankle stability. This also engages all of your leg and core muscles, while increasing calf strength.

Repetition: Complete 7-10 reps, beginning with 7 reps and building up to 10 reps as able. Complete 3 sets.

Good for: Strengthening lower legs for walking and negotiating uneven surfaces.

Movement: **Single Leg Stance with Shoulder Raise**

Flexibility level: **Advanced**

Description:

- Stand with feet shoulder-width apart
- Tighten your tummy muscles to engage your core
- Hold onto a table or chair with one hand
- Lift one leg without bending your knee and raise the opposite arm. Hold for 2-3 seconds, then return to the starting position. Alternate sides.

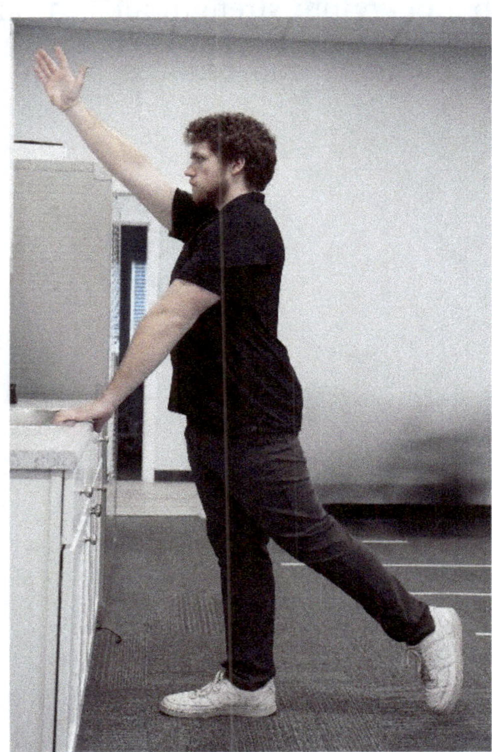

What this does: Activates buttocks and back of thigh muscles while engaging tummy muscles to increase stability.

Repetition: Perform 5-10 reps, beginning with 5 reps and working up to 10 as able. Complete up to 3 sets. Hold each rep for 3-5 seconds before lowering your hips back down to starting position.

Good for: Strengthening your buttocks and back of thighs as well as increasing stability in your abdomen. Increased buttock/glute strength aids in one's ability to walk safely outdoors and reduces strain on the lower back.

Flexibility Exercises

Our muscles adapt over time to the positions in which our bodies function most frequently. It is very common to find muscular tightness accompanying postural problems. The tightness may worsen your posture and limit your ability to engage easily in certain daily activities. Muscles that lack flexibility may become shortened or tight, affecting your progress.

Movement: **Single Knee to Chest Stretch**

Flexibility level: **Beginner**

Description:

- Lie on your back with both legs bent so feet are on the floor
- Draw one leg up, pulling your knee toward your chest, keeping your opposite leg bent (in starting position)
- Hold the stretch for 20-30 seconds, then return to starting position
- Perform the same stretch on the opposite side

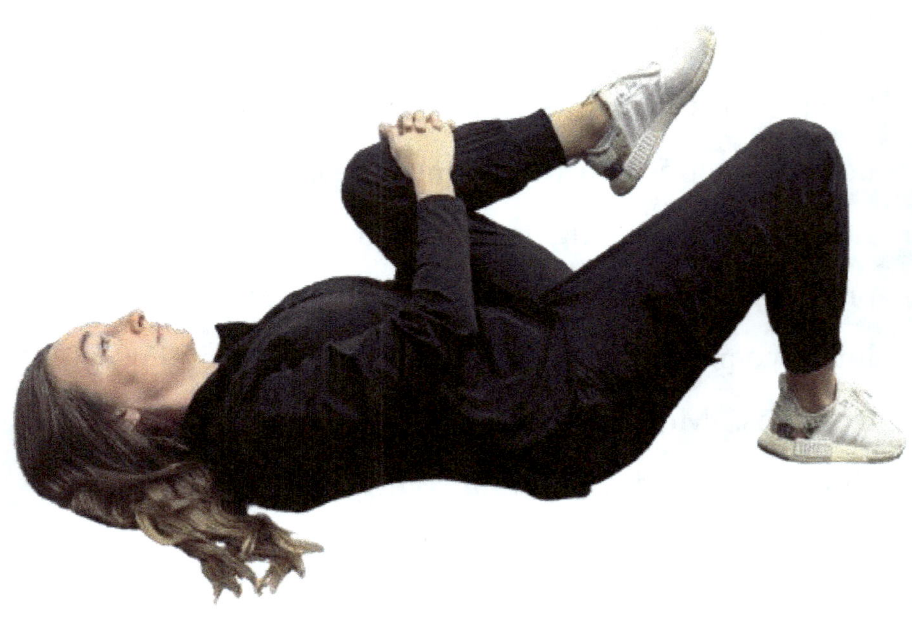

What this does: Stretches the back part of your leg into your buttock. Maintains a neutral spine with opposite leg bent.

Repetition: Perform 3 reps on each side, holding for 20-30 seconds for each rep. Perform twice daily.

Good for: Improving the flexibility in your hamstrings and hips, which will make walking outdoors and climbing up and down stairs easier.

Movement: **Long Sitting Calf Stretch**

Flexibility level: **Beginner**

Description:

- Sit with legs extended straight out in front of you
- Wrap a towel around the bottom of your foot and pull your toes back toward your torso (you should feel a gentle stretch in your calf)
- Hold the stretch for 20-30 seconds, then relax
- Repeat stretch on opposite side

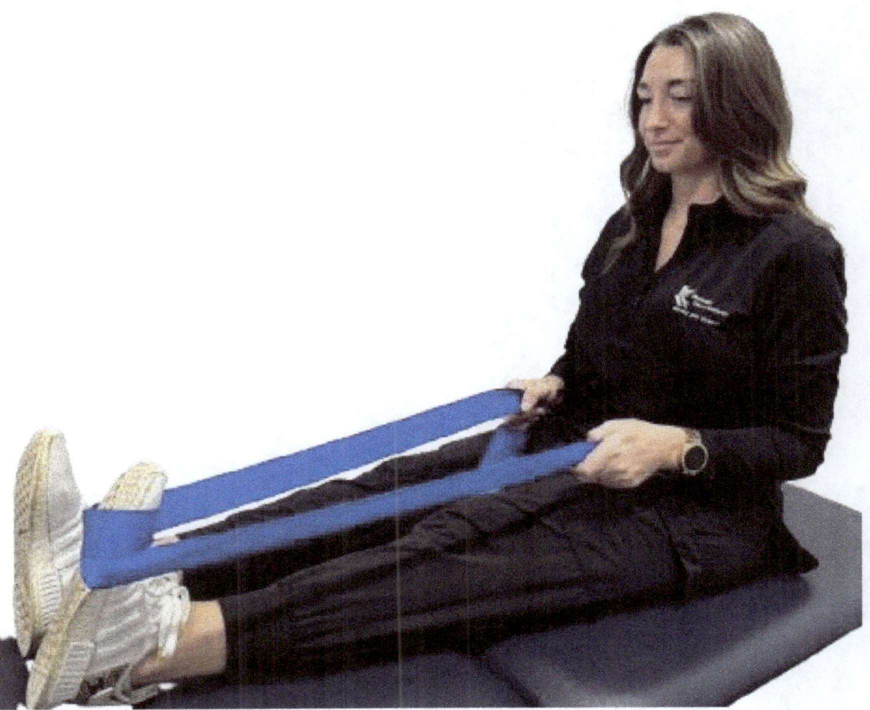

__What this does:__ Stretches lower leg muscles, aiding in greater ankle mobility.

__Repetition:__ Perform 3 reps on each side, holding for 20-30 seconds for each rep. Perform twice daily.

__Good for:__ Improving flexibility in ankles and lower legs, which will help with walking on level, uphill, and uneven surfaces.

Movement: **Supine Hamstring Stretch**

Flexibility level: **Intermediate**

Description:

- Lie on your back with legs bent so feet are flat on the floor
- Place a towel behind one knee and pull your leg in toward your chest so that your hip is at a 90-degree angle
- Gently extend your leg upward until you feel a moderate stretch in the back of your thigh
- Hold the stretch for 20-30 seconds, then return to starting position
- Repeat on opposite side

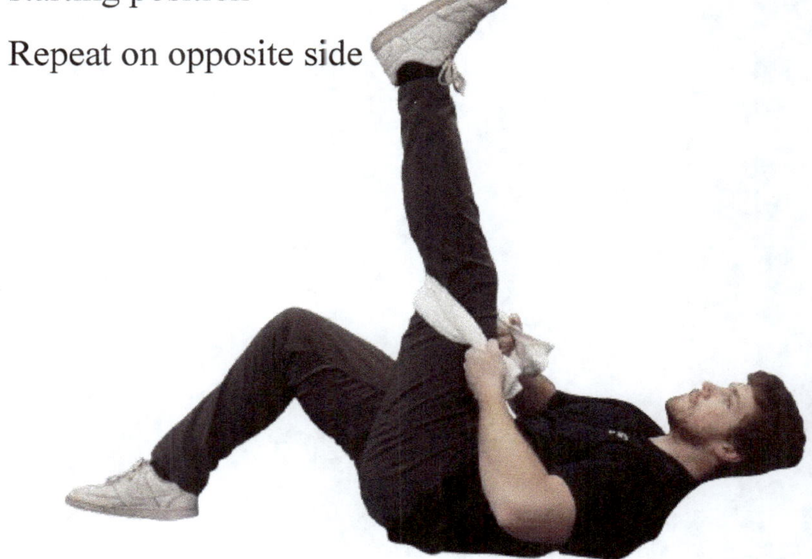

What this does: Stretches hamstring muscles, which helps to improve hip mobility.

Repetition: Perform 3 reps on each side, holding for 20-30 seconds for each rep. Perform twice daily.

Good for: Improving hamstring and hip flexibility to go up and down steps easily, walk faster, get out of your bed and car easier, and get up from a chair.

Movement: **Piriformis Stretch**

Flexibility level: **Intermediate**

Description:

- Lay on your back
- Bend one knee and pull toward opposite shoulder
- Maintain position for 10 seconds, then relax
- Repeat on opposite side

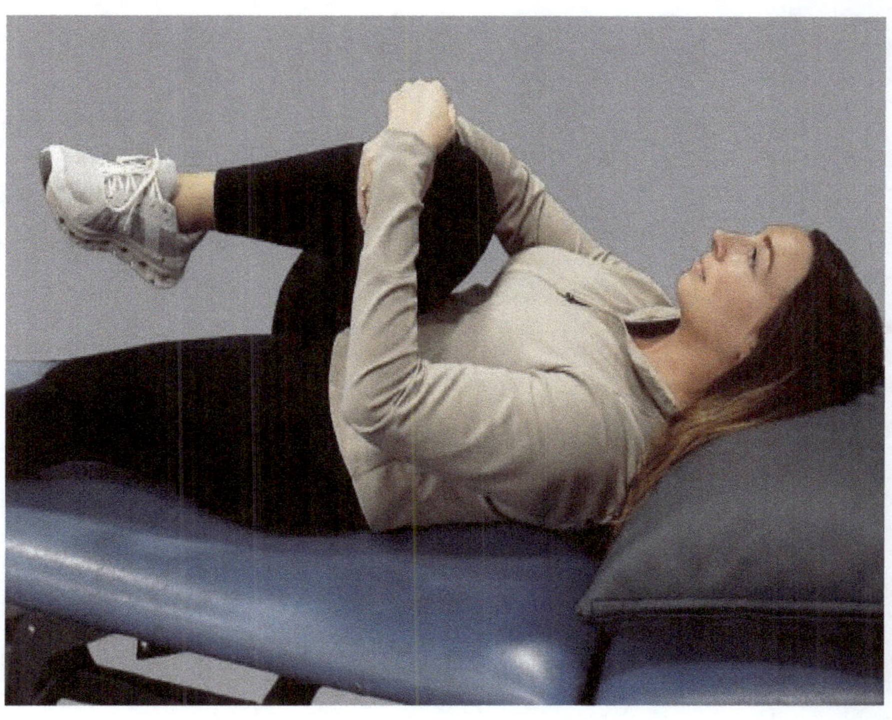

__What this does:__ Stretches the piriformis muscle in your buttocks area.

__Repetition:__ Hold this position for 10 seconds, eventually progressing to 20 seconds. Perform twice daily.

__Good for:__ Improving flexibility in the hip, making going uphill and downhill, getting out of a car, and getting up from the toilet seat easier.

Movement: **Hip Flexor Stretches**

Flexibility level: **Advanced**

Description:

- While holding onto a table or furniture, kneel on one knee with your opposite foot forward. Use a pillow to reduce stress on your knee.
- While kneeling, lean forward and bend your front knee until you feel a stretch along the front of your other hip
- Hold this position for 5-10 seconds
- Return to starting position and repeat on the other side.

What this does: This position will stretch the muscles in the front of your hips.

Repetition: Repeat this movement 10 times per set, once a day. Perform 1-2 sets. Try starting with 1 set and progressing to 2 sets per day.

Good for: Improving flexibility of the hips while walking outdoors (especially for long distances), shopping, and negotiating stairs.

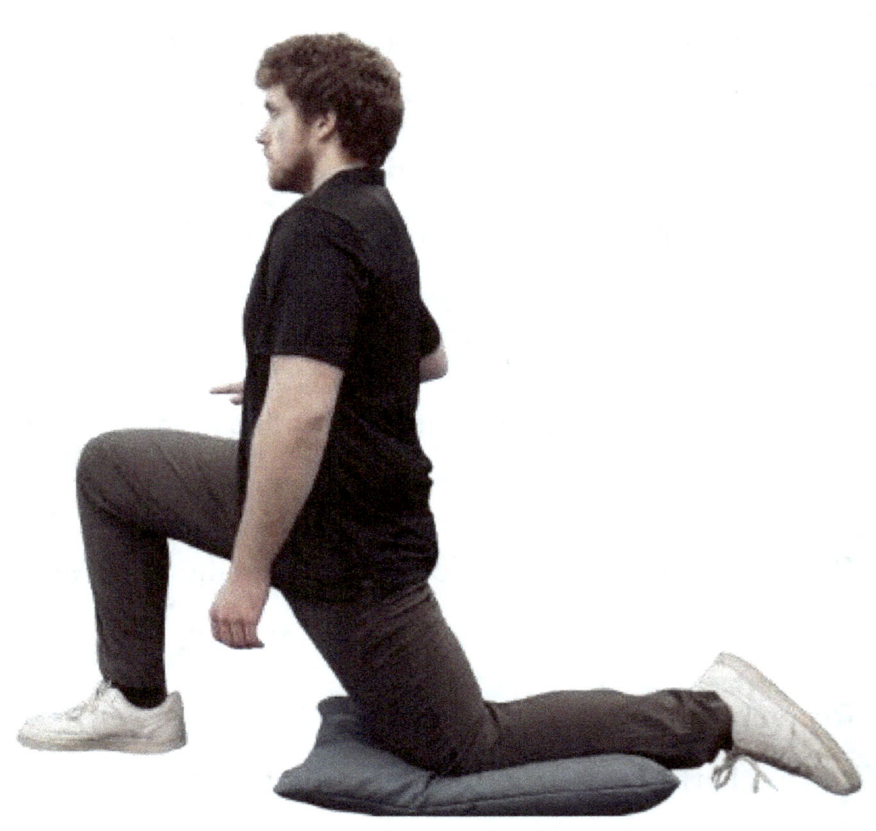

Movement: **IT band (Iliotibial band) Stretches**

Flexibility level: **Advanced**

Description:

- Stand and hold onto a chair with one hand

- Cross one leg behind the other leg

- While using the chair for balance and support, lean forward and away from the crossed leg side. Hold this position for 5-10 seconds

- Return to starting position and repeat on other side.

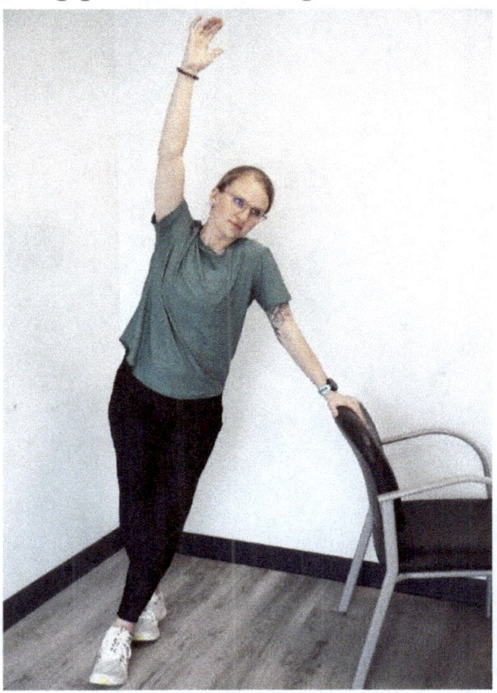

What this does: This will stretch the muscles in the side of your hips and thighs.

Repetition: Repeat this movement 10 times per side, once a day. Perform 1-2 sets. Try starting with 1 set and progressing to 2 sets per day.

Good for: Improving flexibility of hips while walking forward and sideways and increasing ability to sit down in a chair from a standing position.

Balance And Stability Exercises

Balance and stability often decline with aging and become more relevant for those with osteoporosis. Therefore, improving balance and stability is crucial in preventing abnormal posture preventing falls. Incorporation of regular balance exercises will help prevent falls and improve stability in your activities.

Movement: **Two-Foot Balance**

Flexibility level: **Beginner**

Description:

- Stand on a firm surface near a counter or other stationary object for support and safety as needed
- Start with feet shoulder distance apart
- Maintain this position for 30 seconds (without support if possible) to challenge your balance
- Progress by moving your feet closer together, ultimately working toward having your feet together and maintaining this position for 30 seconds without support.

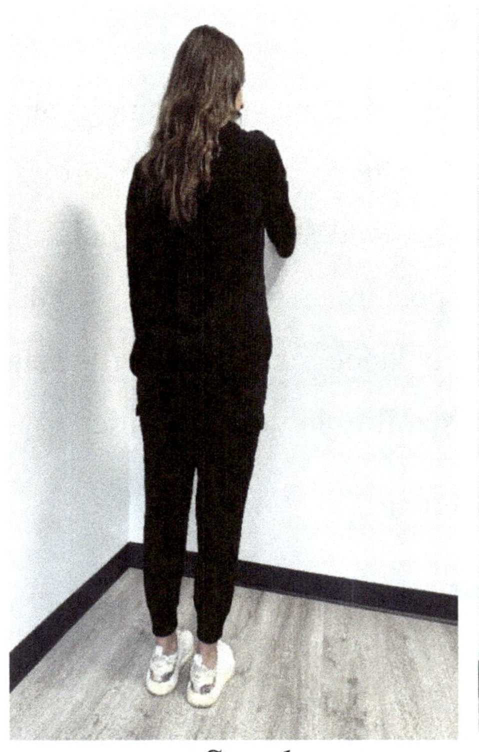 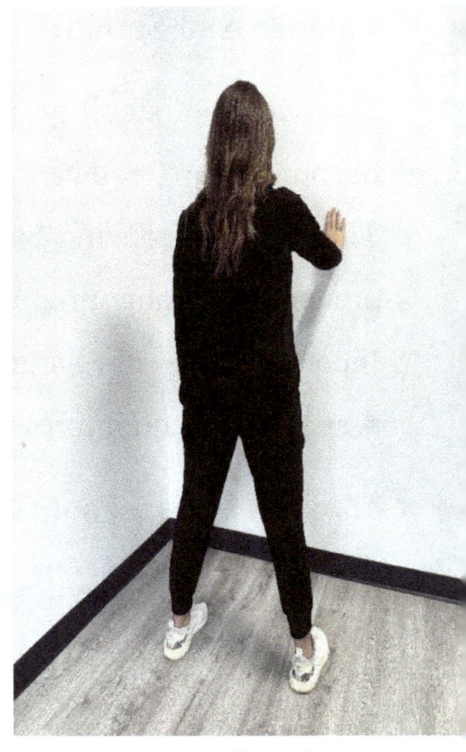

Step 1.   *Step 2*

What this does: Improves your static balance and stability.

Repetition: Hold this position for 30 seconds, repeating 3 times with feet in each position, starting with feet shoulder distance apart and working toward feet together.

Good for: Static balance while brushing teeth or cooking a meal.

Movement: **Side Stepping**

Flexibility level: **Beginner**

Description:

- Stand close to a wall (preferably in a hallway), using one hand to touch the wall for stability
- Lift one foot and take a step sideways
- Walk at least 10 feet in one direction
- Repeat exercise, walking in the opposite direction

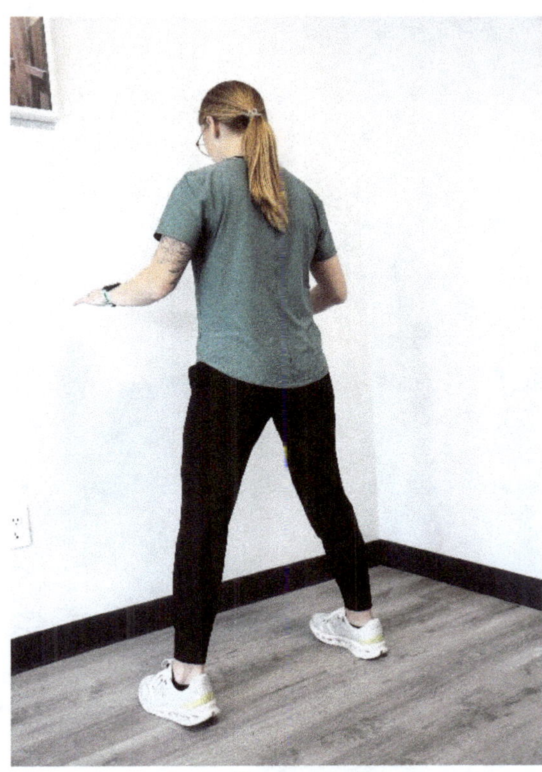

__What this does:__ Works on dynamic balance using a wide base of support.

__Repetition:__ Repeat 5 laps in each direction. You may progress to side-stepping without touching the wall once you feel comfortable.

__Good for:__ Getting your body used to using a wide base of support to improve balance and stability for walking on uneven surfaces like sand, snow, or grass.

Movement: **Tandem Static Balance**

Flexibility level: **Intermediate**

Description:

- Stand on a firm surface near a counter or other stationary object (for safety and support as needed)
- Place one foot in front of the other, with your heel and toe touching
- Maintain this position for 30 seconds, without support, if possible, to challenge balance
- Repeat with opposite leg in front.

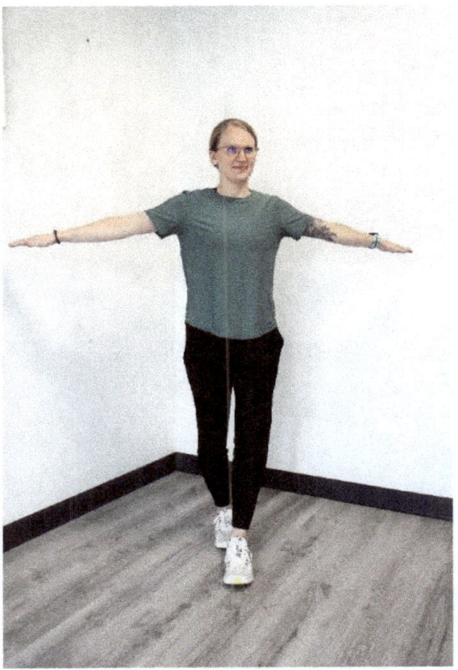

What this does: Works on static balance with a smaller base of support.

Repetition: Hold this position for 30 seconds, then rest. Repeat 3 times with each foot forward. Use a counter for support and safety if necessary (the greater challenge is to perform this exercise without holding on.)

Good for: Improving balance in smaller spaces, such as a hallway or a crowded venue.

Movement: **Toe Stands**

Flexibility level: **Intermediate**

Description:

- Stand on a firm surface near a counter, wall, or other stationary object (for safety and support as needed)
- Place your feet 1 foot apart, placing fingers on the counter or wall for balance
- Raise both heels and maintain this position for 10 seconds
- Progress by not using fingers for balance.

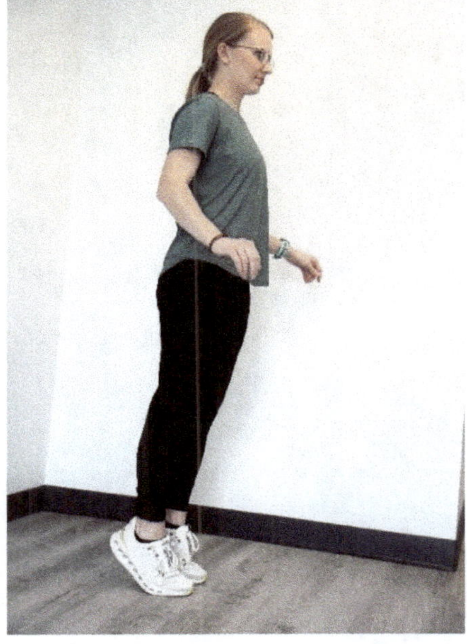

What this does: Works on static balance with a smaller base of support.

Repetition: Hold this position for 10 seconds, then rest. Repeat 10 times, once a day. You may use a counter for support and safety, but the greater challenge is to perform these exercises without holding on.

Good for: Improving balance in smaller spaces, such as a hallway, standing in a moving bus, or walking around a crowded venue.

Movement: **Single Leg Balance**

Flexibility level: **Advanced**

Description:

- Stand on a firm surface near a counter or other stationary object (for safety and support as needed)
- Stand on one foot, with opposite foot at ankle or knee height (knee height will be more of a challenge)
- Engage abdominal muscles for greater stability
- Balance on one leg for 10 seconds, progressing to 30 seconds as able
- Use a counter for support and safety as needed (the greatest challenge is to perform this exercise without any support)
- Repeat on opposite side.

What this does: Works on single-leg balance, hip strength, and hip and core stability.

Repetition: Hold this position for 10 seconds, progressing to 30 seconds as able. Repeat 3 times on each side, once daily.

Good for: Improving the single-leg balance needed to negotiate stairs or curbs, and also improves one's ability to dress oneself.

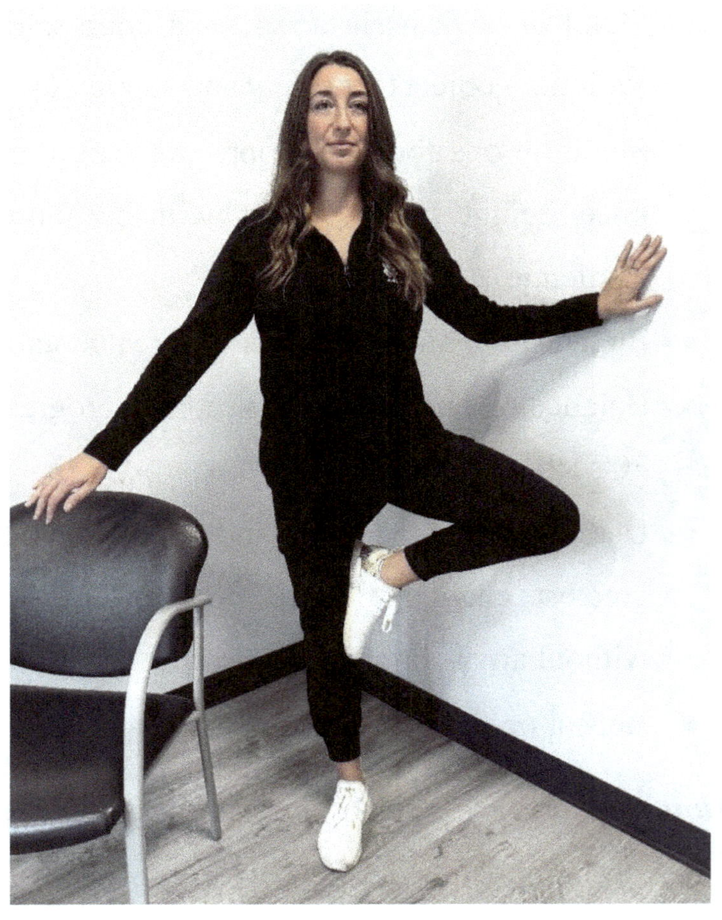

Movement: **Tandem Walking**

Flexibility level: **Advanced**

Description:

- Stand close to a wall

- Engage abdominal muscles for greater stability

- Place one foot in front of the other in a heel-toe pattern

- Walk forward slowly with arms raised to sides for stability

- Walk for at least 10-15 feet.

What this does: Works on improving your dynamic leg balance, weight-bearing ability, and hip and core stability. This also helps with increasing bone density.

Repetition: Turn around and walk in the opposite direction. Repeat 10 laps, once a day.

Good for: Preventing falls by improving balance while walking on even or uneven surfaces.

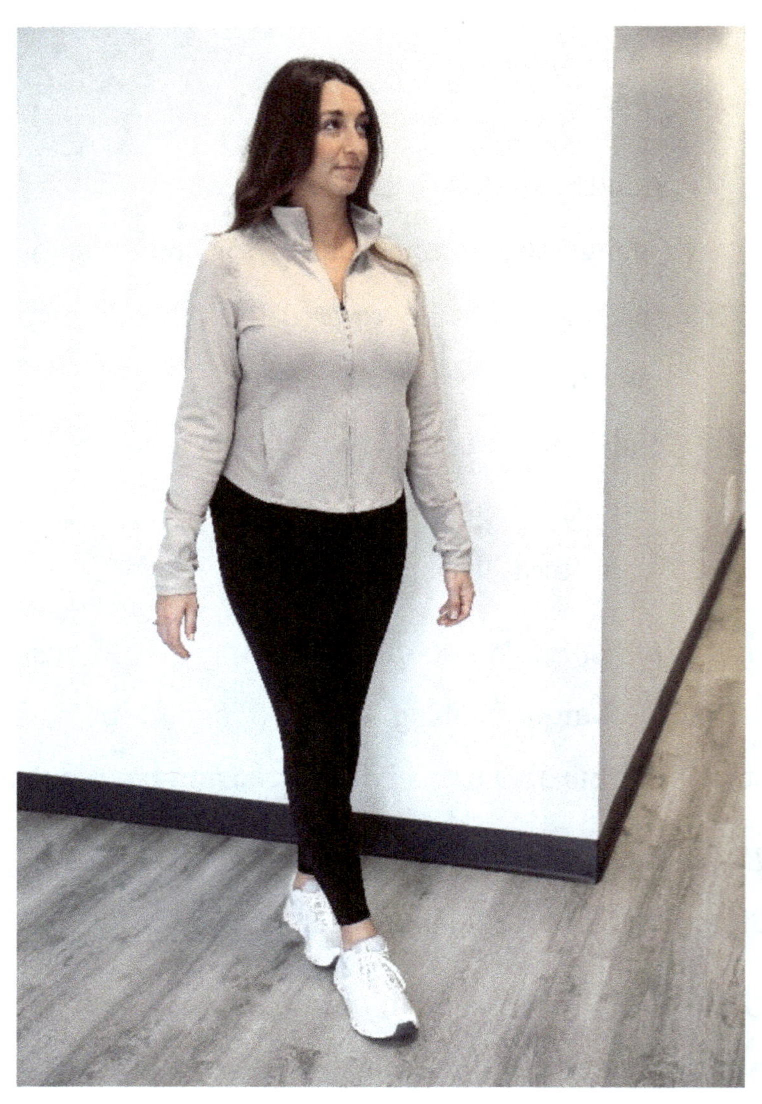

Chapter 5

The Nutrition And Exercise Plan In Action

Introduction

Now that you have an idea of the significance of a well-balanced diet and the importance of exercises for preventing bone loss and regaining bone strength, let's focus on an actionable nutrition and exercise plan for each experience level that will help you improve the health of your bones.

How To Use This Chapter

Following an exercise plan while you are suffering from osteoporosis might seem scary and overwhelming. Yet, the information provided in this manual will help ease your fears and calm your mind, in addition to boosting your bone health. It is important to remember, however, that we won't see an immediate effect from these exercises. Instead, you will notice slow and steady improvements as you adopt the plan.

For the best outcome, I recommend that you continue to do these exercises regularly with the proper food intake. Breaking the exercise routine at any point before the completion period is not advisable, as it may fail to provide the expected results. You should plan on spending approximately one month on each level and should be able to finish the program over the course of three months. However, if you have increased lower back pain or have any other illness, this may take longer. If your pain increases or it feels like you are fatigued faster, stop the exercises immediately and contact your medical provider.

Sidebar: Keeping A Journal

Maintaining a workout journal is one of the easiest and most productive ways to track your progress over time. Jotting down the level of exercises performed, number of repetitions done, and intake of consumed diet will help you understand your current bone strength and progress of bone health. Filling out a journal both before and after carrying out your exercise plan each day helps track mood patterns and improve your mental health. Journaling your exercises also helps you stay motivated and positive while transitioning into a new lifestyle with improved bone health. So,start journaling today and feel proud of your achievement!

Table 5.1: Osteoporosis Workout Journaling

DATE	EXERCISE LEVEL	DIET INTAKE	COMMENTS	RECOMMENDATIONS

What Level Am I On?

You can use the chart below to help determine with which exercise level you should begin. If you feel like you do not fit into any of the levels below, you can choose exercises that can be done either sitting or lying down as listed in chapter 4. If you still feel overwhelmed or physically limited, you may benefit from getting help from a trained physical therapist.

Easy	Moderate	Challenging
• Able to stand for at least 5 minutes without lower back pain • Able to lift 3-4 pounds (about the weight of a half-gallon of milk) • Need to	• Able to stand for 10-15 minutes without lower back pain • Able to lift 7-8 pounds (about the weight of a gallon of milk) • Mild loss of balance	• Able to stand for 30 minutes without lower back pain • Able to lift weights above 10 pounds • No loss

hold onto an object to avoid loss of balance • Experience shortness of breath after a few reps	• Intermittent shortness of breath	of balance • No shortness of breath

The Easy Level

The easy (or beginner-level) type of osteoporosis exercises are meant to enhance the bones of people with poor bone health. These easy-level exercises, along with the intake of essential bone nutrients, promote the development of stronger bones, thereby helping to improve your lifestyle and health conditions. The easy-level exercises will help you improve strength and stability with standing activities and household chores.

Nutrition Intake

As mentioned earlier, to prevent bone loss and build strong bones, I recommend you incorporate foods that are rich in calcium, protein, vitamin D, vitamin C, vitamin K, magnesium, and zinc. Here is an example of a healthy meal plan recommended by the American Dietetic Association and the International Osteoporosis Foundation:

Breakfast:

- Orange juice fortified with calcium and vitamin D
- Whole grain cereal fortified with vitamin D
- Skim milk

Lunch:

- Extra-lean ground beef on a whole grain bun with non-fat American cheese, 1 piece of lettuce, or 2 slices of red tomato
- Green leafy salad with 1 hard-boiled egg and low-calorie dressing
- Skim milk

Snack:

- Orange

Dinner:

- Chicken breast
- Broccoli
- Strawberries with whipped topping

Recommended Shopping List

Your shopping list may include:

- Fat-free or low-fat milk products such as milk, yogurt, cheese, or plant-based milks such as soy or almond milk
- Calcium-fortified orange juice
- Calcium-fortified cereal
- Green leafy vegetables such as spinach, kale, and broccoli
- Seafoods such as salmon, tuna, and sardines
- Meat products such as ground beef and chicken

I strongly suggest you look for varieties of fruits and vegetables that are of different colors. The more colors, the better! To reduce your salt intake, check the nutrition label for the sodium level and only purchase foods with low levels of sodium. This is especially important to check if you are purchasing canned vegetables. Similarly, if you are going for frozen vegetables, be sure to choose one with no or less butter or cream sauce.

Sidebar: Ramping Up

If you are new to an osteoporosis exercise plan, or if you are back on track after a break, I recommend that you start your exercises at a slow pace by doing them for only 15 minutes a day, 2-3 times a week, before gradually progressing to doing the exercises for around 30 minutes per day, at least 3 times per week. Doing the exercises this way makes the arm and leg muscles work harder which, over time, helps in the development of stronger bones and helps to increase bone density.

Sequence:

Movement 1:

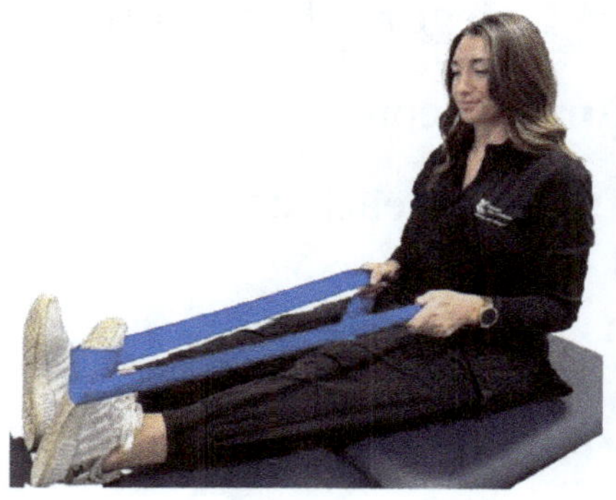

- **Movement:** Supine Calf Stretches

- **Exercise Category:** Flexibility

- **Hold For:** 5 seconds

- **Repeat:** 7 times each day

Movement 2:

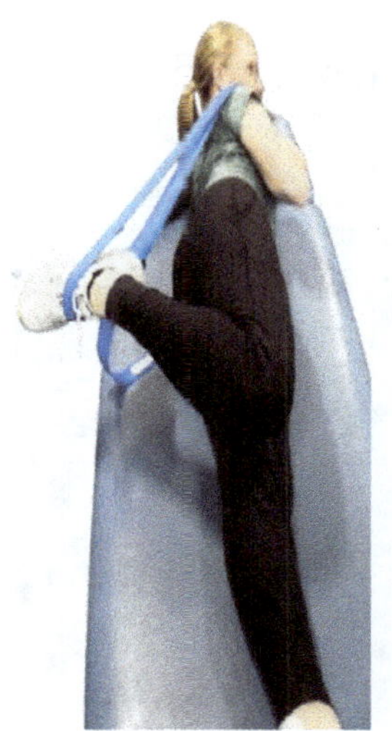

- **Movement:** Side Lying Quadricep Stretch

- **Exercise Category:** Flexibility

- **Hold For:** 5 seconds

- **Repeat:** 7 times each day

Movement 3:

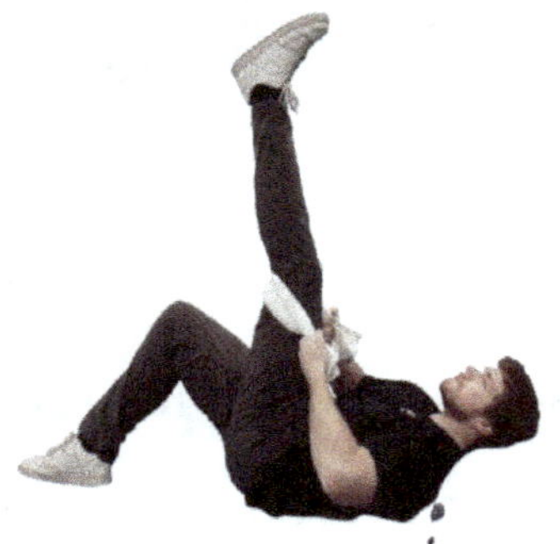

- **Movement:** Supine Hamstring Stretches

- **Exercise Category:** Flexibility

- **Hold For:** 5 seconds

- **Repeat:** 7 times each day

Movement 4:

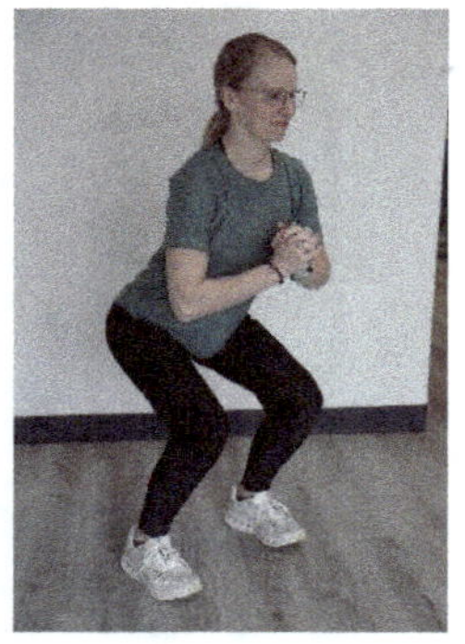

- **Movement:** Standing Partial Squats (1A)

- **Exercise Category:** Strengthening

- **Hold For:** 1-2 seconds

- **Repeat:** 7-10 times per set. Perform three sets each day

Movement 5:

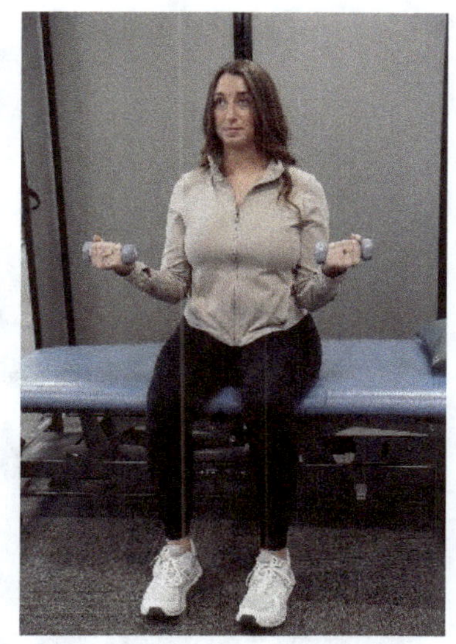

- **Movement:** Bicep Curls

- **Exercise Category:** Strengthening

- **Hold For:** 1-2 seconds

- **Repeat:** 7-10 times per set. Perform three sets each day

Movement 6:

- **Movement:** Side Stepping

- **Exercise Category:** Weight Bearing

- **Hold For:** n/a

- **Repeat:** Step 5 times in each direction, twice a day

Movement 7:

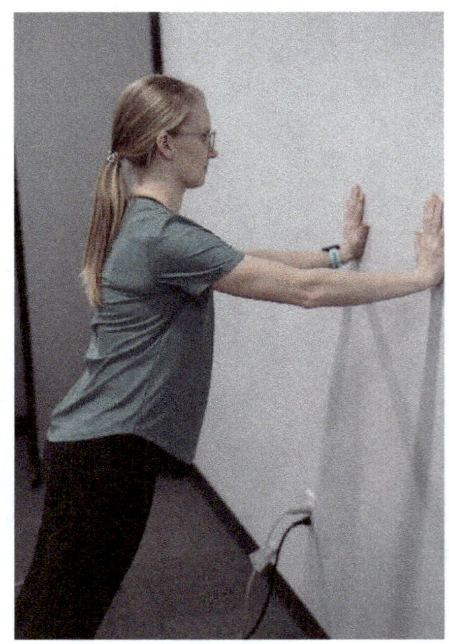

- **Movement:** Wall Push Ups

- **Exercise Category:** Weight Bearing

- **Hold For:** 1 second

- **Repeat:** 7-10 times each set. Perform 3 sets total each day

Movement 8:

- **Movement:** Two-Foot Balance
- **Exercise Category:** Balance and Stability
- **Hold For:** 30 seconds
- **Repeat:** 3 times with each foot, for each position

Movement 9:

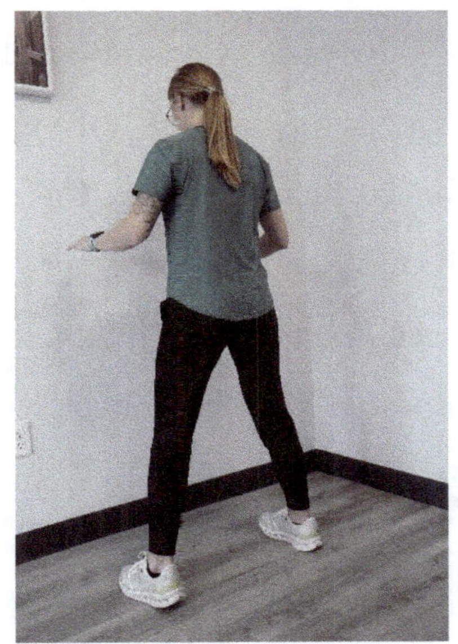

- **Movement:** Walking Sideways
- **Exercise Category:** Balance and Stability
- **Hold For:** n/a
- **Repeat:** Move 10 feet in each direction. Perform 5 sets in each direction

Sidebar: Time To Heal

Osteoporosis is a serious condition that requires a long time to heal. Trying to perform all the osteoporosis exercises right away does not work. Your body needs time to repair and recover from your health condition. Similarly, exercising very vigorously only increases the risk of fractures. Therefore, it is important to do the right exercises at a slow pace. Consuming the right diet and nutrients (as per the advice of your doctor) and performing the correct exercises for no more than 15 minutes each day can boost your healing process. Continuing these habits over a long period of time heals and further improves your bone health.

Moderate Level

Moderate (or intermediate) exercises strengthen your body's core, hip, and knee muscles, increase your bone density, and improve your stability and ability to balance and perform various tasks and activities. These exercises should be done at a faster pace than the easy-level exercises and supplemented with a proper diet plan that incorporates additional bone nutrients into your diet.

The moderate-level exercises should help you with different activities of daily living like dressing, cooking, short-distance walking, and improving your balance while helping to improve your bone density.

=Nutrition Intake

Simply completing these exercises (without implementing a proper meal plan) will not maximize your healing process. Along with the right exercise plan, adopting a well-balanced diet, complete with bone nutrients that help form strong bones, aids in preventing osteoporosis. As you transition from beginner to intermediate-level exercises, it is essential that you increase your intake of nutrients in order to promote your bone health and increase your bone density. Here is an example of a healthy meal plan recommended by the American Dietetic Association and the International Osteoporosis Foundation:

Breakfast:

- Scrambled tofu with bell peppers and spinach

- Oven-roasted potatoes with skim milk and American shredded cheese

Lunch:

- Whole wheat wrap with red pepper hummus, grated carrot, and tomatoes
- An apple or banana

Snack:

- Fruit smoothie blended with low-fat skim milk or yogurt

Dinner:

- Grilled chicken sautéed with zucchini, asparagus, and mushrooms

Your shopping list may include:

- Milk products such as Vitamin D milk, yogurt, cheese, or plant-based milks such as soy or almond milk
- Green beans, collard greens, kale, broccoli, and/or oranges (which are rich in calcium)
- Calcium-fortified breads and cereals

- Whole grains, oatmeal, and almonds

- Seafoods such as salmon, tuna, or oysters

- Turkey (dark meat), chicken, and eggs

Sequence:

Movement 1:

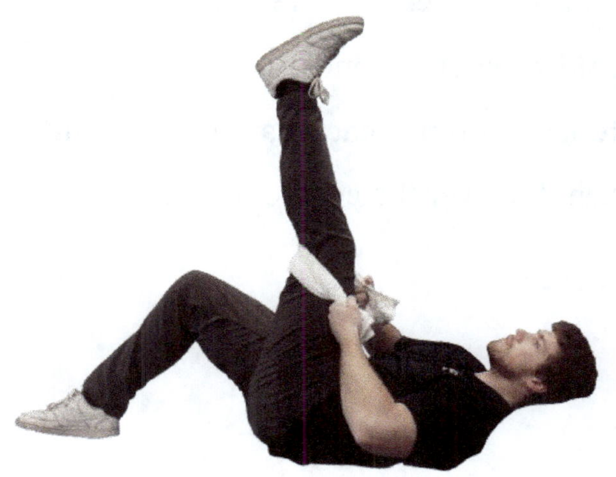

- **Movement:** Supine Hamstring Stretch (2C)

- **Exercise Category:** Flexibility

- **Hold For:** 20-30 seconds

- **Repeat:** 5 times each day

Movement 2:

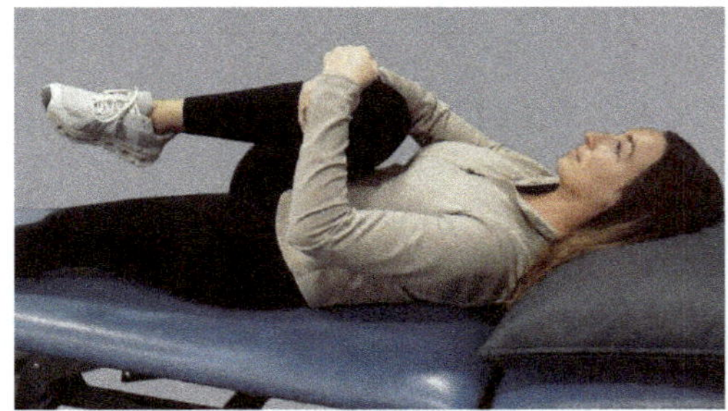

- **Movement:** Piriformis Stretch

- **Exercise Category:** Flexibility

- **Hold For:** 10 seconds

- **Repeat:** 5 times each day, progressing to 7 times each day over the course of one week

Movement 3:

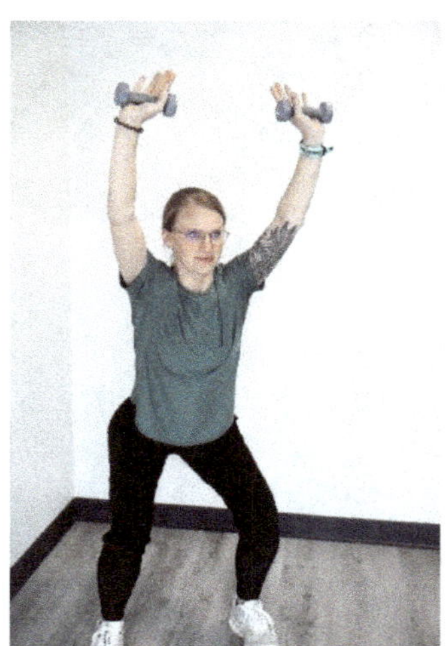

- **Movement:** Partial Squat Position Shoulder Press with Dumbbell

- **Exercise Category:** Strengthening
- **Hold For:** 1-2 seconds
- **Repeat:** 7-10 times each set. Perform 3 sets each day

Movement 4:

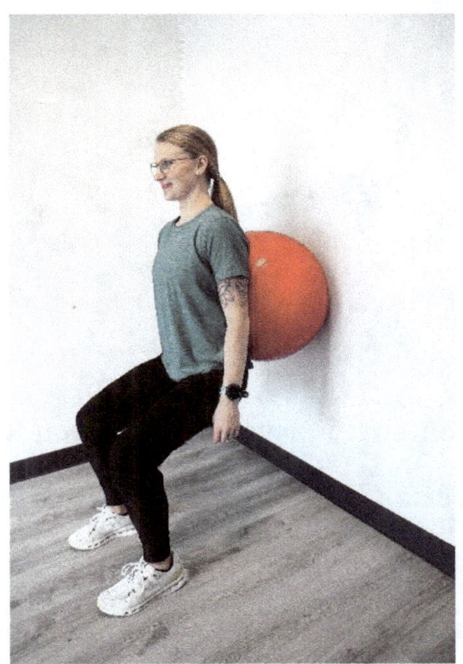

- **Movement:** Partial Squats with Ball Behind Back
- **Exercise Category:** Strengthening
- **Hold For:** 1-2 seconds
- **Repeat:** 7-10 times per set, perform 3 sets each day

Movement 5:

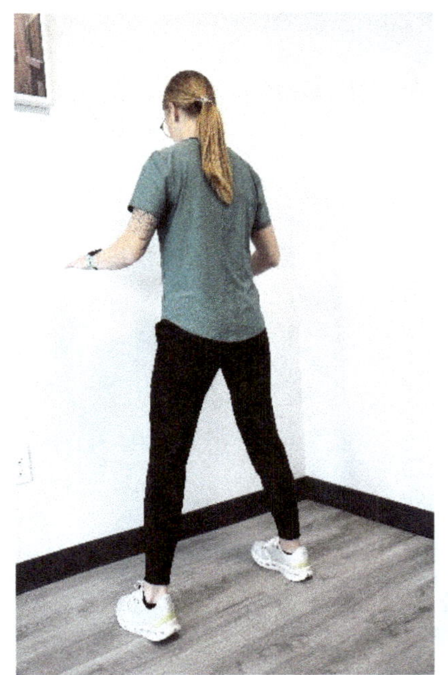 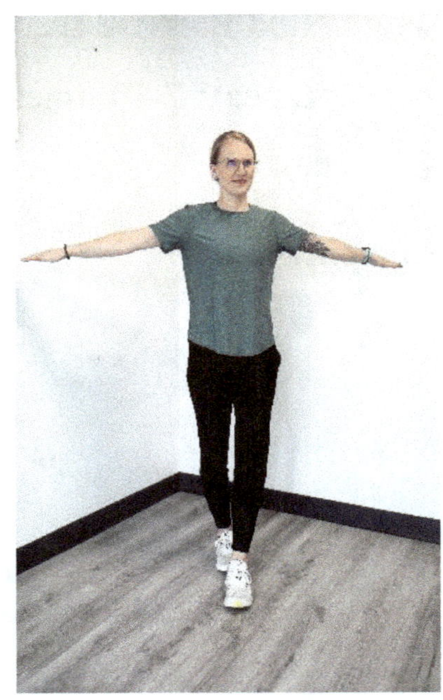

- **Movement:** Forward and Lateral Step Ups

- **Exercise Category:** Weight Bearing

- **Hold For:** n/a

- **Repeat:** 7 times each (right foot forward, right foot sideways, left foot forward, and left foot sideways). Start with 7 reps for each leg and build up to 10 reps on each side over the course of one week.

Movement 6:

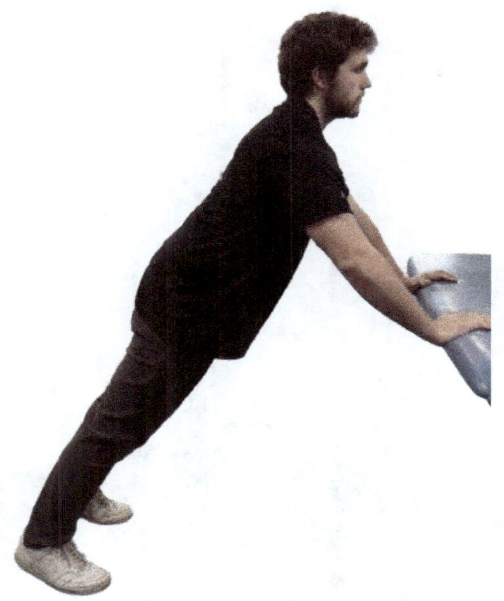

- **Movement:** Table Level Plank

- **Exercise Category:** Weight Bearing

- **Hold For:** 10-30 seconds

- **Repeat:** 7-10 reps per set, 3 sets total per day

Movement 7:

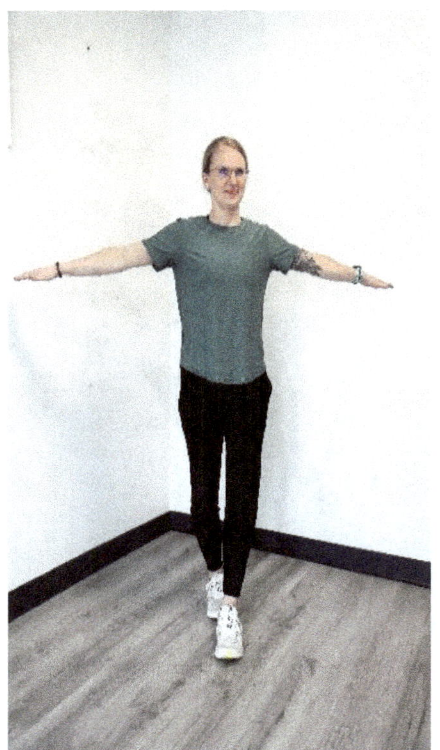

- **Movement:** Tandem Static Balance

- **Exercise Category:** Balance and Stability

- **Hold For:** 30 seconds

- **Repeat:** 3 times with each foot, for each position

Movement 8:

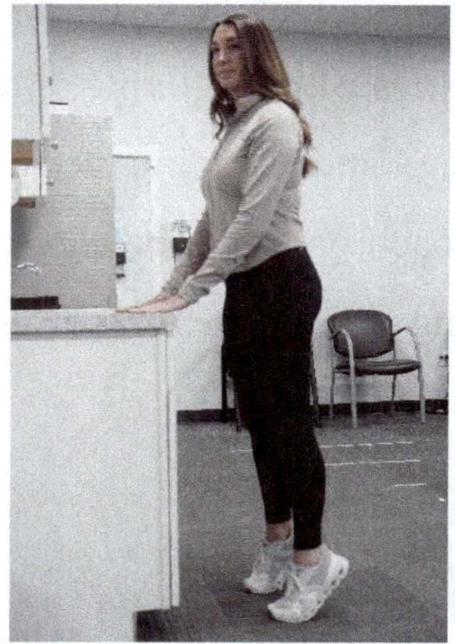

- **Movement:** Toe Stands

- **Exercise Category:** Balance and Stability

- **Hold For:** 10 seconds, slowly building up to 20 seconds

- **Repeat:** 10 times per day

The Challenging Level

The advanced (or challenging) level of exercises stimulates the overall bone health and should be carried out in sets of 7-10 repetitions. Start with one set and slowly progress to two sets per day. Remember not to rush or exercise too vigorously, as it may worsen your bone health condition. This level of exercise will help you tolerate activities of daily living, and prevent falls, prolonged walking, and standing activities. With the right, gentle approach, you will be sure to achieve your goal of enhancing the growth and development of stronger bones.

Nutrition Intake

Stepping into the advanced level of exercise requires an updated diet plan. Here is an example of a healthy meal plan recommended by the American Dietetic Association and the International Osteoporosis Foundation:

Breakfast:

- Omelet or quiche with desired vegetables
- Calcium-fortified juice or skim milk

Lunch:

- Salmon burger on whole grain bun
- Mashed potatoes

Snack:

- Rice or milk pudding

Dinner:

- Nachos topped with avocado, kidney beans, and low-fat cheese
- Greek salad with feta cheese

Recommended Shopping List

Your shopping list may include:

- Vitamin D-fortified milk, plant-based milk, or calcium-fortified orange juice
- Cheese and yogurt
- Prunes, raisins, cantaloupe, figs, and citrus fruits such as grapefruit
- Winter squash, broccoli, spinach, edamame, or sweet potatoes
- Green leafy vegetables such as turnip greens, collard greens, spinach, kale, and broccoli
- Seafoods such as swordfish, canned or fresh tuna fish, and sardines

- Meat products such as ground chicken, turkey (dark meat), and beef

Movement 1:

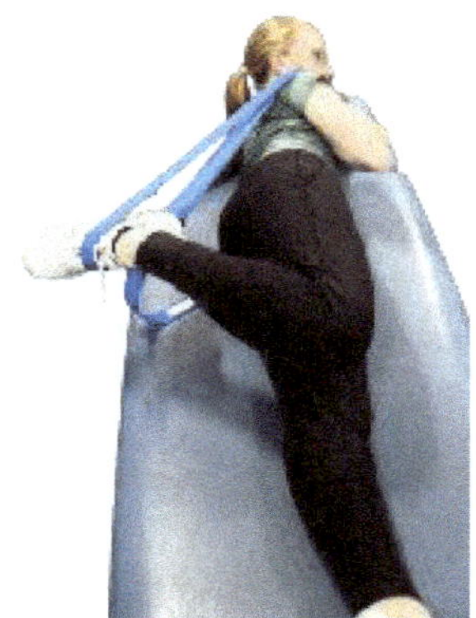

- **Movement:** Side Lying Quadricep Stretch (2A)
- **Exercise Category:** Flexibility
- **Hold For:** 5-10 seconds
- **Repeat:** 10 times each day. Progress to 2 sets a day over the course of two weeks

Movement 2:

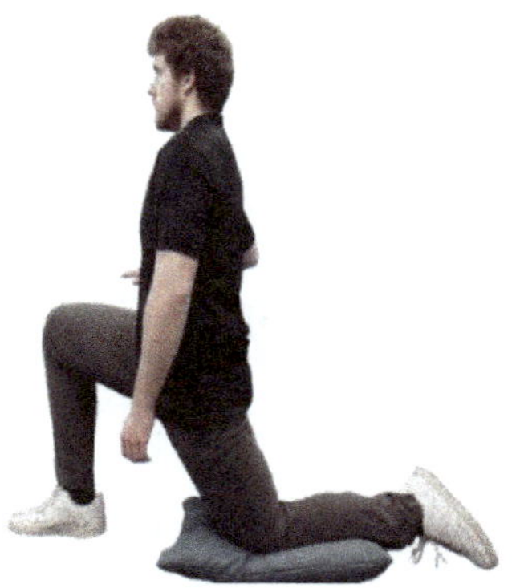

- **Movement:** Hip Flexor Stretches (2D)

- **Exercise Category:** Flexibility

- **Hold For:** 10 seconds, progressing to 20 seconds over the course of one week

- **Repeat:** 5 times each day

Movement 3:

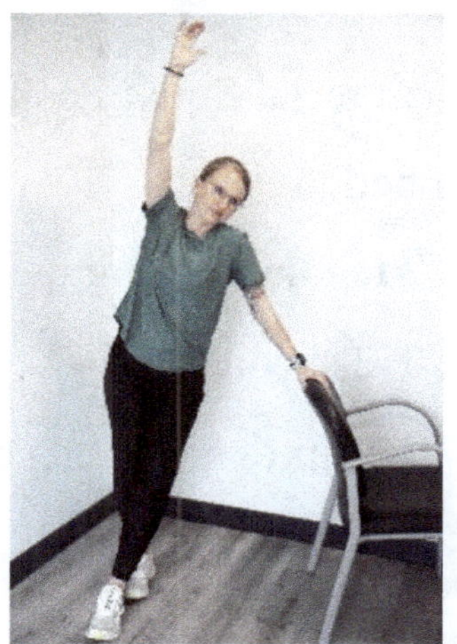

- **Movement:** IT Band Stretches (2E)

- **Exercise Category:** Flexibility

- **Hold For:** 5-10 seconds

- **Repeat:** 10 times each day, one set per day. Progress to 2 sets per day over the course of one week

Movement 4:

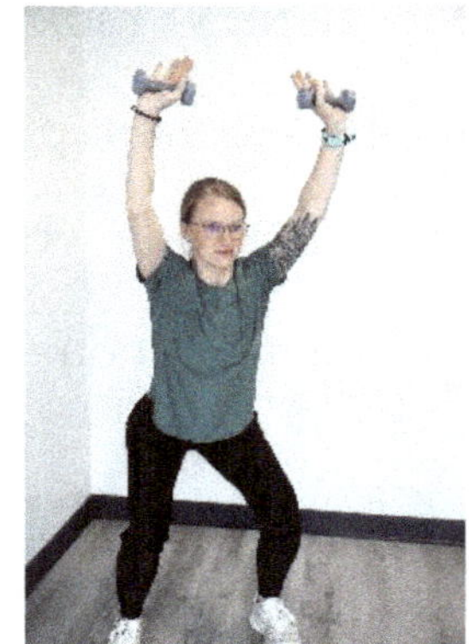

- **Movement:** Partial Squat Position Shoulder Press with Dumbbell (1C)
- **Exercise Category:** Strengthening
- **Hold For:** 1-2 seconds
- **Repeat:** 7-10 times per set, perform 3 sets each day

Movement 5:

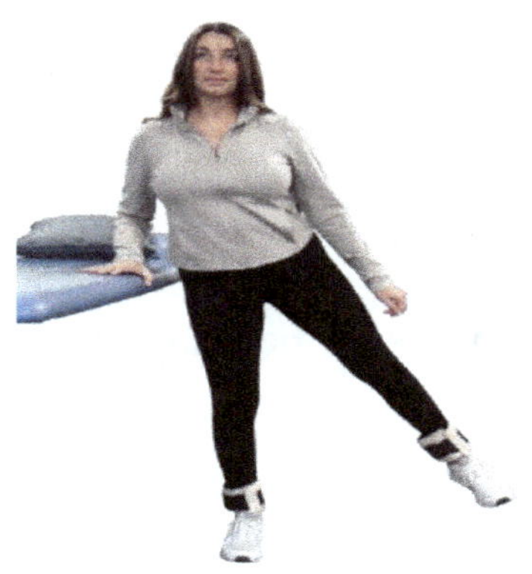

- **Movement:** Sideways Leg Lift

- **Exercise Category:** Strengthening

- **Hold For:** 1-2 seconds, with 2–3-pound ankle weights on each side

- **Repeat:** 7-10 times per set. Perform 3 sets each day. Try starting with 7 reps and progressing to 10 reps per set

Movement 6:

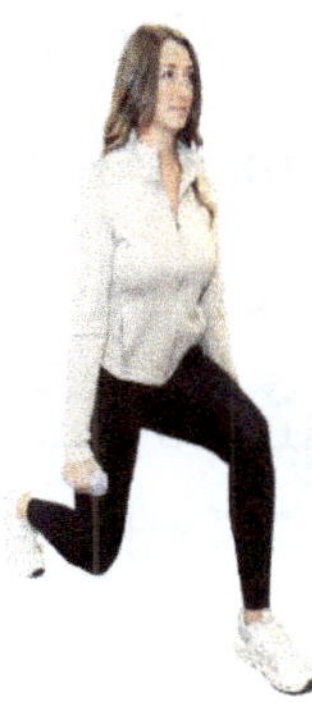

- **Movement:** Forward Lunges with Weight (1F)

- **Exercise Category:** Weight Bearing

- **Hold For:** n/a

- **Repeat:** 7-10 times per set leading with your right foot and 7-10 times per set leading with your left foot. Try starting with 7 reps and progressing to 10 reps per set

Movement 7:

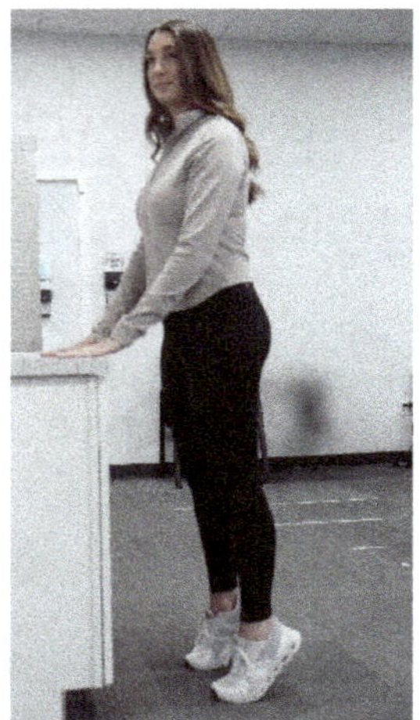

- **Movement:** Calf/Heel Raises

- **Exercise Category:** Weight Bearing

- **Hold For:** 1-2 seconds

- **Repeat:** 7-10 times each set. Perform 3 sets total each day

Movement 8:

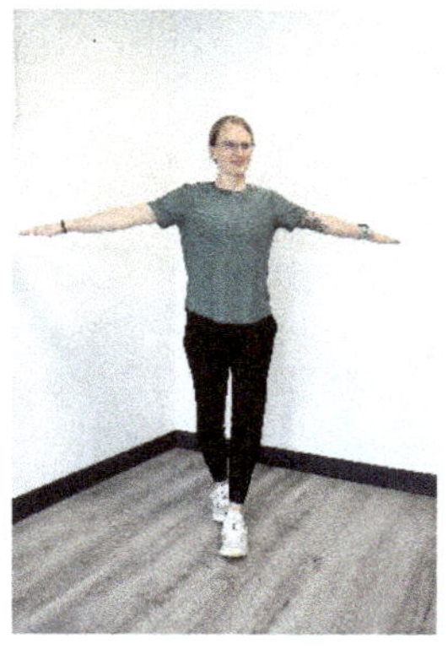

- **Movement:** Single Leg Balance (4E)

- **Exercise Category:** Balance and Stability

- **Hold For:** 10 seconds, building up to 30 seconds

- **Repeat:** 3 times per day, leading with each side

Movement 9:

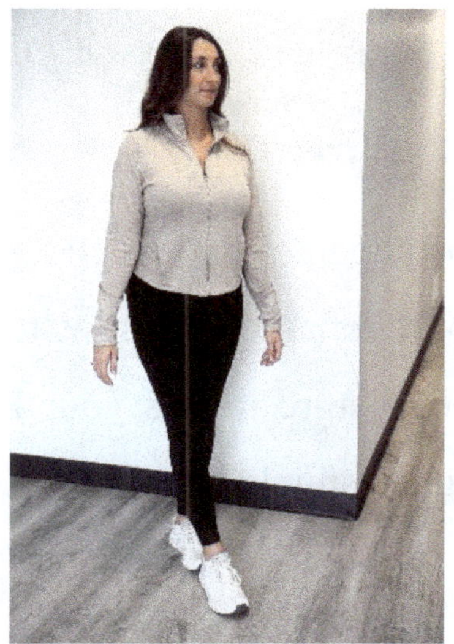

- **Movement:** Tandem Walking (4F)

- **Exercise Category:** Balance and Stability

- **Hold For:** n/a

- **Repeat:** Move 10-15 feet in each direction. Perform 10 laps each day.

Posture And Osteoporosis

Healthy posture goes a long way toward maintaining good spinal and bone health, especially in people with osteoporosis. Osteoporosis is a bone condition that weakens them and makes your bones break easily. These risks are not only made worse when combined with poor posture but are also improved and controlled by good posture.

The Logic Of Posture:

Posture is the arrangement in which a person holds their body during stationary poses, sitting, or moving positions. Good posture means your bones, joints, and muscles are aligned snugly and in position, which further minimizes the amount of unnecessary stress on these body parts!

Impact Of Poor Posture

Kyphosis (increased forward curvature of the thoracic spine) due to poor posture not only changes the natural alignment of the spine but can also create spinal compression, which in turn increases the risk of compressed vertebrae. When you cough, sneeze, or reach for something, poor postural alignment can cause spinal column micro-trauma.

Resource Impairment Of Balance:

Poor posture throws us out of whack, affecting our balance and stability. This makes falls even more severe for anyone with osteoporosis.

Muscle Weakness And Fatigue:

Prolonged poor posture may also lead to muscle weakness, making us more prone to osteoporotic bones.

Benefits Of Good Posture

Decreased Fracture Risk: Good posture means that all bones are well aligned and, hence, safer from any external impact.

Better Balance: Strong postural alignment holds better balance for coordinated movement, reducing the risk of falls.

Improved Breathing and Digestion: An aligned spine and torso combination will maximize lung capacity and digestion, both of which are vital for overall health.

Good Posture Maintenance Tricks

Adjustments in the workplace: Adopting a neutral posture, with lower back support when sitting and computer screens at eye level, which makes you look straight without tilting your neck down, can help.

Exercise-strengthening exercises for the muscles of the core, back, and legs, especially yoga and Pilates practices.

Mindfulness and breaks: Pay attention to your posture throughout the day. Stand, stretch, and align your body for a few minutes every hour or so.

In summary, good posture is essential for managing osteoporosis. In addition to preventing fractures, poor alignment can negatively impact the quality of life by destroying healthy spinal muscles.

These exercises will successfully improve and maintain your posture. You can perform them at any time during the day, and they do not need to be completed alongside the movements listed in Chapter 4.

Postures and positions to avoid

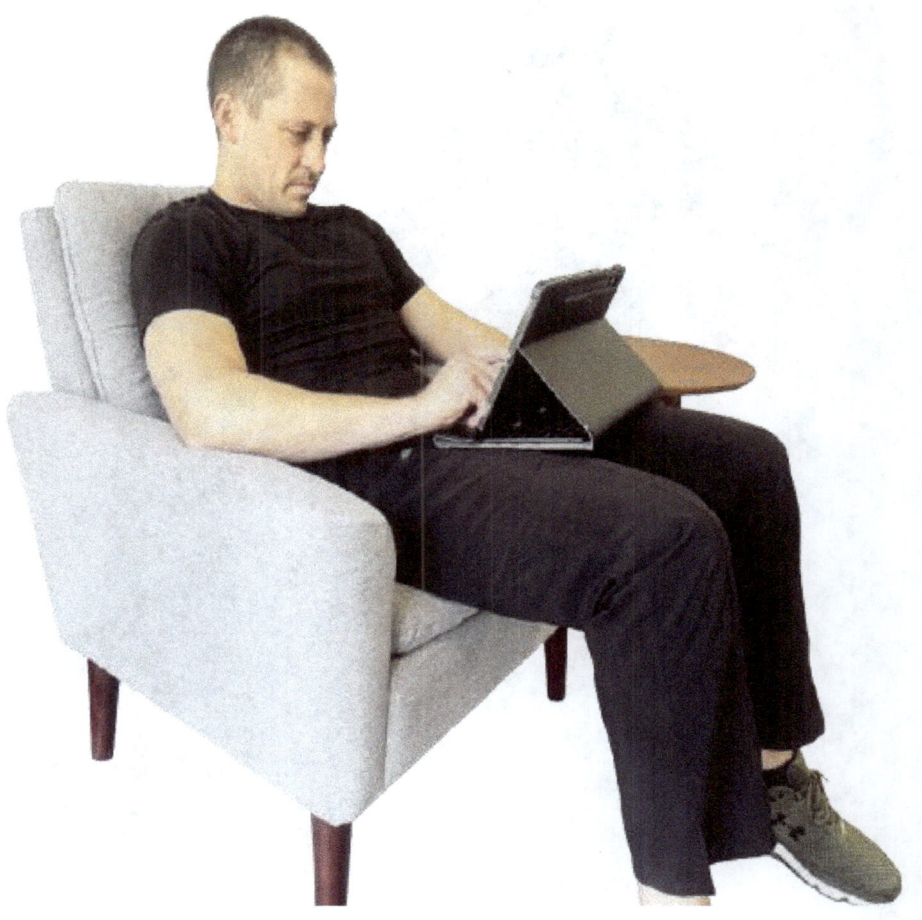

Correct posture

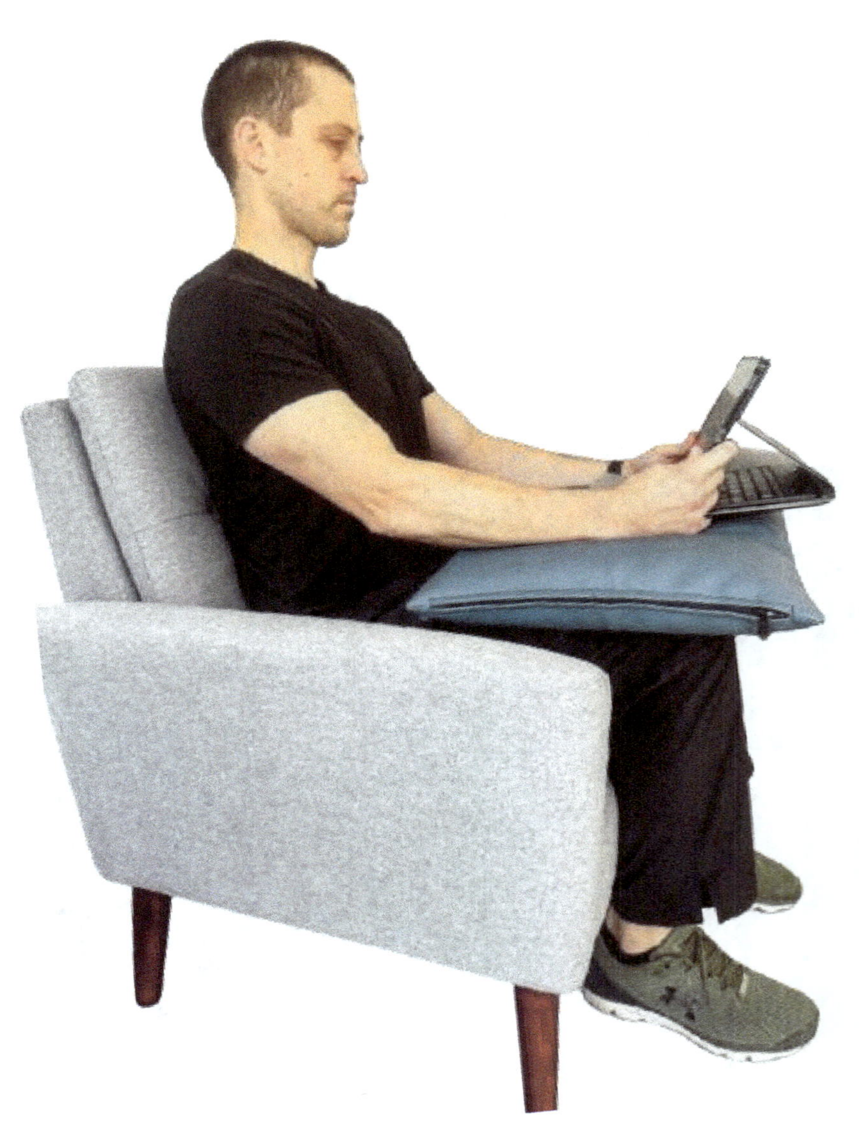

Postures and positions to avoid

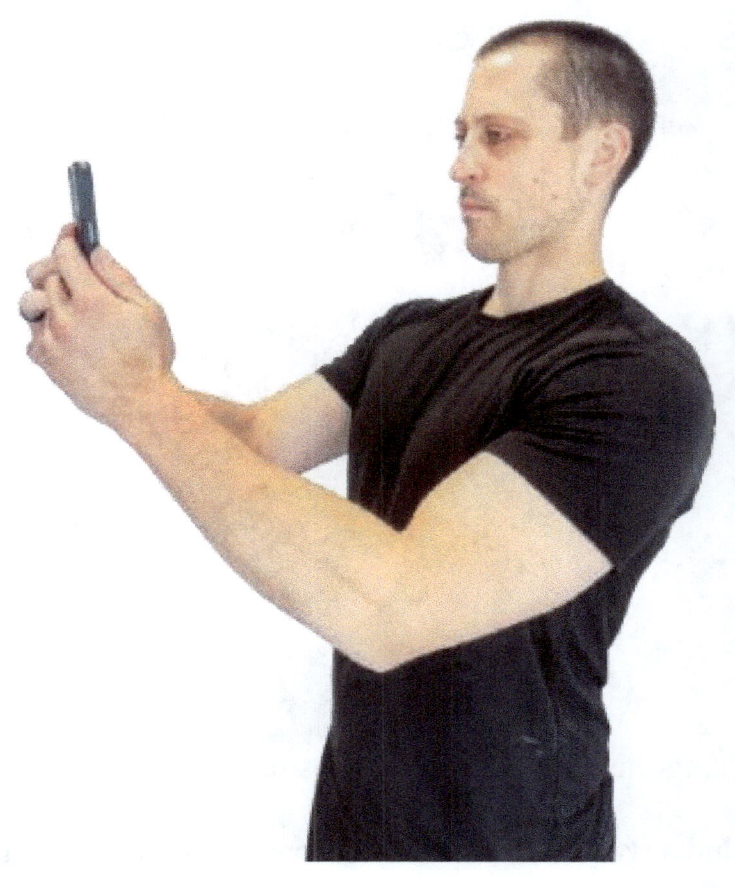

Correct posture

Posture Corrective Exercises

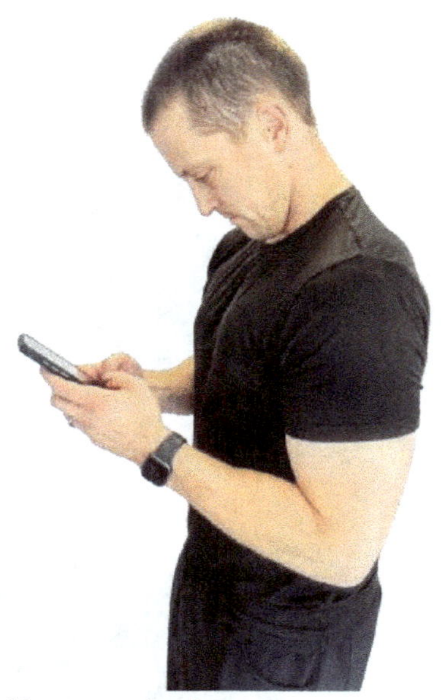

Using the wall to optimize posture

Find a wall and position your back against the wall. Push your head, shoulders, and

buttocks toward the wall. Now, tuck your tummy in. Hold for 2-3 seconds. Repeat 5-7 times.

Scapular Squeezes

Squeeze your shoulder blades together making sure the shoulders are down.

The Anti-Sloucher Exercise

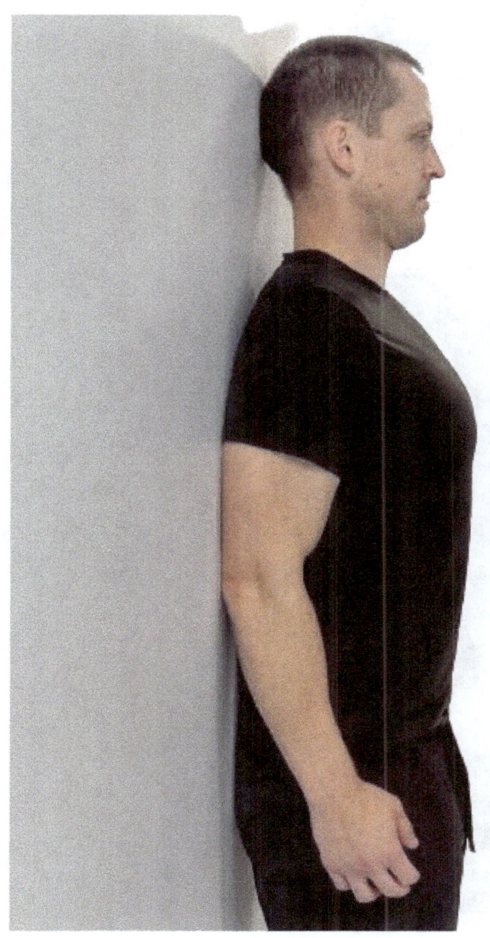

Step 1:

Squeeze the shoulder blades and tuck the chin.

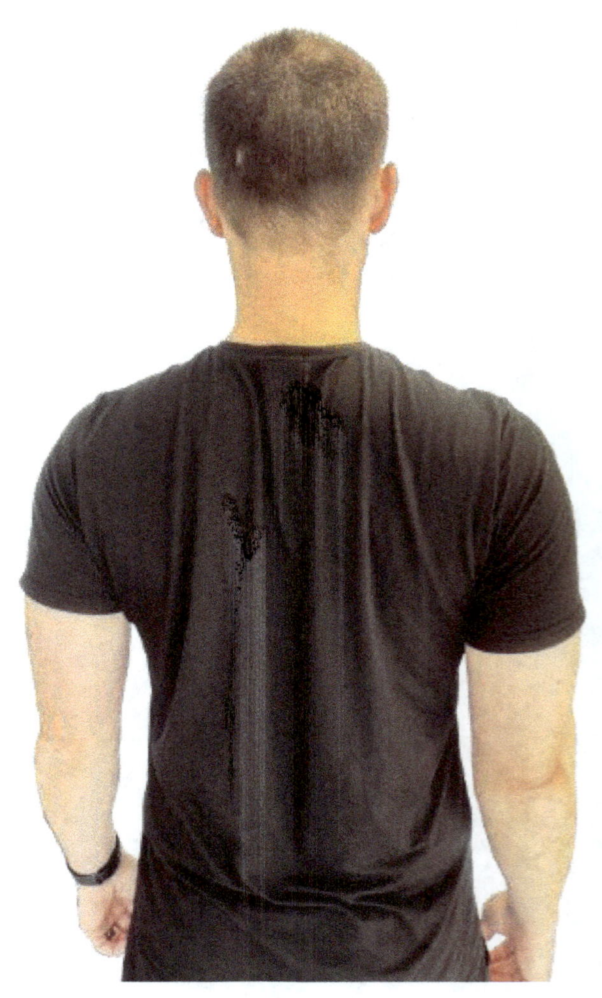

Step 2:

Once you feel comfortable doing the above exercise, lift the clasped handbehind you. Hold for 3-5 sec and relax. Repeated ten times

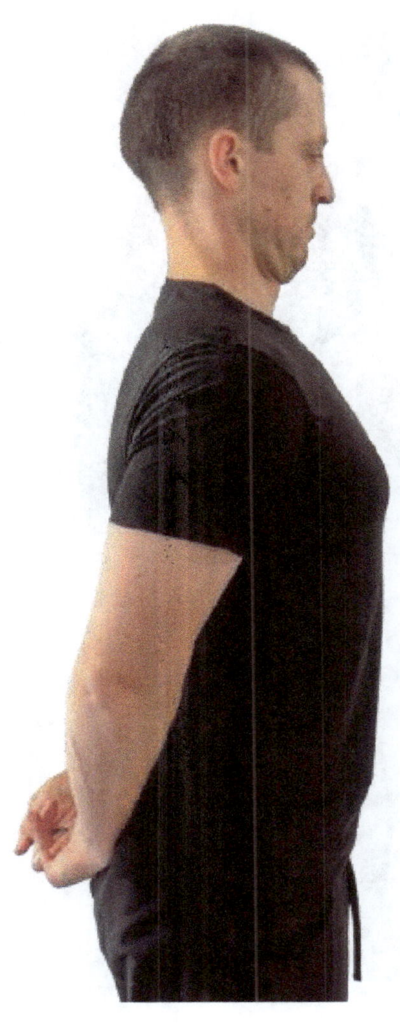

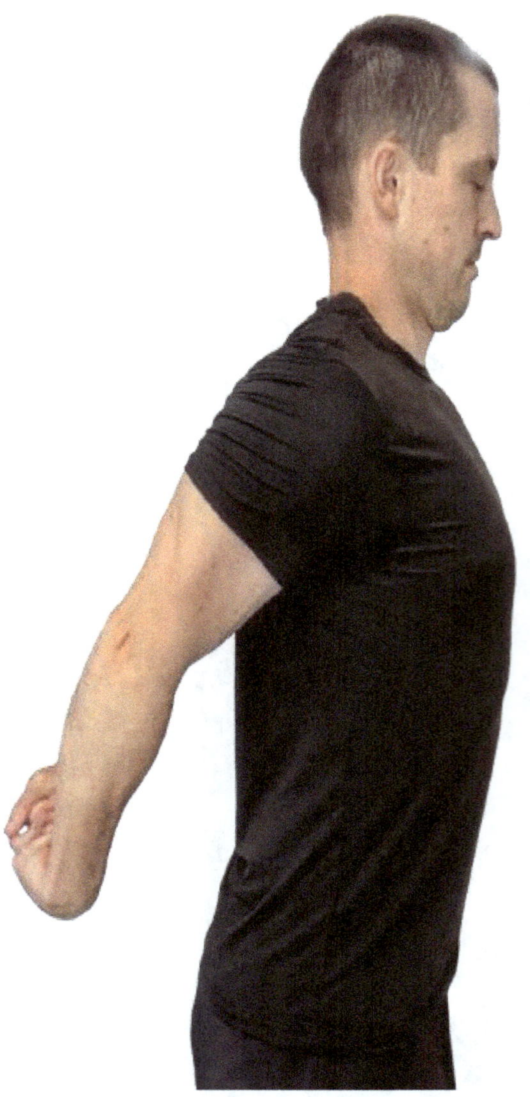

As shown in the picture below, take an elastic resistance band and pull to both sides while squeezing the shoulder blades.

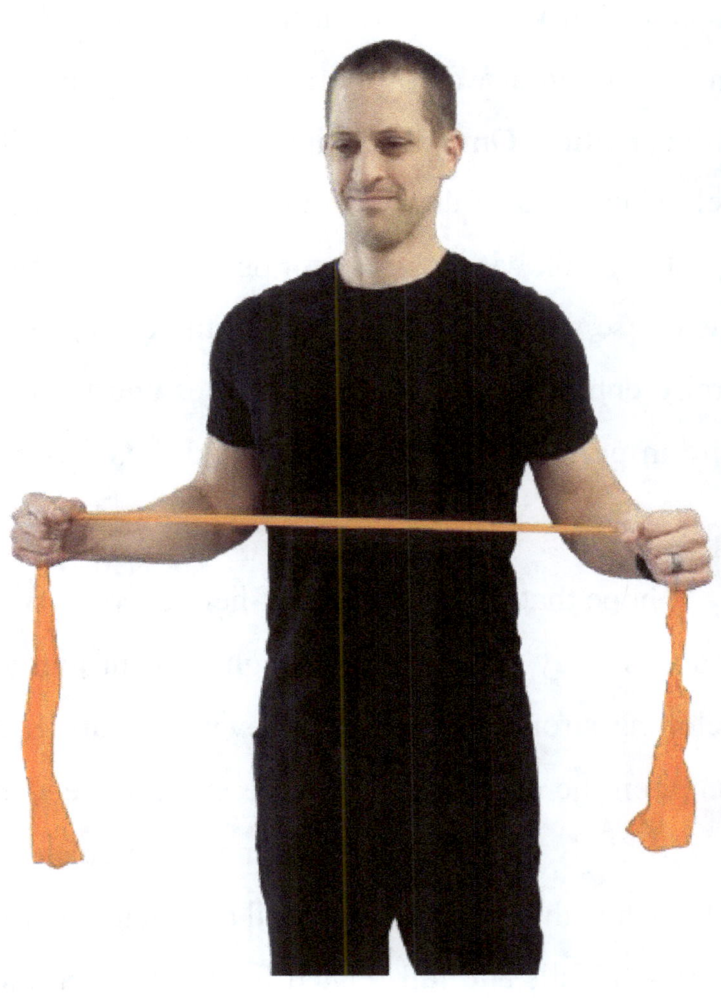

Wrapping Up

Now that we have discussed each phase of this exercise plan, I strongly suggest that you continue doing these exercises every day while following the appropriate diet plan. Consuming the right nutrients helps you long term to enjoy your way of living with an improved bone health condition. Only discontinue these exercises if you develop any kind of discomfort or pain, in which case I suggest you talk with your doctor before continuing with the exercise plan. Various research studies suggest that exercise enhances the strength of bones and the quality of life in people with osteoporosis and those with poor bone health.

I hope that this at-home self-help exercise manual will act as a key and aid you throughout your journey of developing stronger bones and preventing further bone loss. Upon the completion of these exercise sequences, you will likely notice an improvement in your stability and bone health. By doing so, it will also help you reduce your risk of falls and fall-related fractures. Even though consuming foods with the proper bone nutrients and adopting the correct exercise plan enhances bone health, I strongly recommend that you consult with your doctor before you begin your journey through this osteoporosis self-help exercise manual.

I wholeheartedly wish all my readers a happy life with good health and the best healing. Thank you.

References

American Bone Health. (2020, December 14). *ABH Fracture Risk Calculator*. American Bone Health. https://americanbonehealth.org/calculator/

Brooke-Wavell, K., Skelton, D. A., Barker, K. L., Clark, E. M., De Biase, S., Arnold, S., Paskins, Z., Robinson, K. R., Lewis, R. M., Tobias, J. H., Ward, K. A., Whitney, J., & Leyland, S. (2022). Strong, steady and straight: UK consensus statement on physical activity and exercise for osteoporosis. *British Journal of Sports Medicine, 56*(15), 837–846. https://doi.org/10.1136/bjsports-2021-104634. Epub ahead of print. PMID: 35577538; PMCID: PMC9304091.

Genuis, S. J., & Bouchard, T. P. (2012). Combination of Micronutrients for Bone (COMB) Study: Bone Density after Micronutrient Intervention. *Journal of Environmental and Public Health, 2012*, 1–10. https://doi.org/10.1155/2012/354151

NOF. (2018, September 4). *Bone Density Test, Osteoporosis Screening & T-score Interpretation.* National Osteoporosis Foundation.

https://www.nof.org/patients/diagnosis-information/bone-density-examtesting/

NOF. (2020, April 2). *Calcium/Vitamin D Requirements, Recommended Foods & Supplements.* National Osteoporosis Foundation.

https://www.nof.org/patients/treatment/calciumvitamin-d/

Stanghelle, B., Bentzen, H., Giangregorio, L., *et al. (2018)* Effect of a resistance and balance exercise programme for women with osteoporosis and vertebral fracture: study protocol for a randomized controlled trial. *BMC Musculoskeletal Disorders* **19,** 100 (2018) https://doi.org/10.1186/s12891-018-2021-y

Resources

1. National Osteoporosis Foundation
https://www.nof.org/patients/

2. Patient education: Osteoporosis prevention and treatment (Beyond the Basics)
https://www.uptodate.com/contents/osteoporosis-prevention-and-treatment-beyond-the-basics

3. Ortho Info- osteoporosis
https://orthoinfo.aaos.org/globalassets/pdfs/osteoporosis.pdf

4. For nutrition information for osteoporosis
https://www.osteoporosis.foundation/health-professionals/prevention/nutrition

5. More exercises for osteoporosis
www.rehabspecialistsmi.com

Where To Get Exercise Equipment?

Most of the needed accessories, such as therapeutic resistance bands, dumbbells, and exercise gym balls, can be obtained from local stores like Walmart, Target, Five Below, or any sporting goods store.

A variety of online stores also carry these items and are readily available on websites like

1. www. amazon.com,
2. www.walmart.com
3. www.target.com